# The BodyEnergy™
# LONGEVITY
## PRESCRIPTION

# The BodyEnergy™
# LONGEVITY
## PRESCRIPTION

How CranioSacral Therapy Helps
Prevent Alzheimer's and Dementia
While Improving the Quality
of Your Life

Michael Morgan, LMT, CST-D

The BodyEnergy Longevity Prescription
*How CranioSacral Therapy Helps Prevent Alzheimer's and Dementia*
*While Improving the Quality of Your Life*
Copyright © 2014 by Michael Morgan LMT, CST-D

Body Energy Company
306 E. Jefferson Avenue
Fairfield, IA 52556

Cover Design and title page by George Foster
Interior Design by Bill Groetzinger

ISBN 978-0-578-14820-5

Printed in the United States of America

# DEDICATION

To Dr. John Upledger—creator of the vision of CranioSacral Therapy, a global inspiration, friend and mentor. To all my students and clients who have been my best teachers.

# ACKNOWLEDGEMENTS

As someone once said, it takes a village to raise a child. In the case of writing a book, my experience is that it requires an entire community to create a finished product.

In that light, I would like to acknowledge the following in my community:

First of foremost, my mentor Dr. John Upledger for his pioneering work on CranioSacral Therapy, and specifically his insights into inflammation and the pathogenic response. Thanks to Nancy Swisher for her inspiration about what it takes to write and edit a book, Dr. Tim Hutton for his precise scientific critique and generous overview of the work, Ms. Tamara Watt for her unflagging and tireless dedication to this project and her keen eye, and especially an acknowledgment to experienced editor Will Mathes for making this a much more readable and enjoyable book. Thanks also to Rebekah Walker and Brittany Crawford for so many hours of research and support. All of you have played an integral part in bringing this book to life.

Inspiration for the book and the video project that accompanies this work goes to Jeffrey Smith, as well as John Kremer for guiding this effort from the beginning, and Tami Goldstein for showing what is possible when bringing your dream to fruition. A special nod to George Foster, a national expert in creating compelling book covers, and to Bill Groetzinger for adding the final graphic touches to this work.

Thanks also for the ongoing support of John Matthew Upledger, who plays a key role in keeping the vital work of CranioSacral Therapy alive in the world. As part of my cranial work, Suzanne Scurlock Durana, Emily Klik, Avadhan Larson and the entire Upledger staff have provided ongoing support and encouragement.

Also great thanks to my functional medicine doctor Karyn Shanks MD who is a true pioneer in the medical field. Great thanks also to my friends Richard Sims, John and Taren Stob, Denese Gallagher and Carla and Duncan Brown. To all my clients and students, who have been the real teachers of Longevity. Without my introduction to Alzheimer's and Dementia by my stepmother Edith Morgan and sister in law Carol Morgan this book would never have been written. Thank you for the inspiration to change the world with a different approach to treating this disease.

# FOREWORD

Alzheimer's dementia is one of the great tragedies of the 21st century and a problem we are learning is preventable. It is one of the many signs we as a culture, as a result of our diets and lifestyle habits, are already a train running off the tracks. Alzheimer's is just one of many manifestations of the great collision between our genetic predispositions, the environment and the state of our bodies exposed to the standard American diet and lifestyle. It is often heralded as "Type 3 Diabetes," because of its apparent link to inflammation and insulin resistance.

The good news Michael Morgan eloquently delivers is that there is hope! We now know we are not slaves to our genetics. We know the expression of our genes and the state of our health can be changed, when we tend to the very basics of self-care, through good food and healthy living.

Michael shows us how we can heal as individuals and as a society, and that Alzheimer's does not have to be our legacy to future generations. We know what to do. There are profound ways we can ameliorate the suffering of our elders and their caregivers, who are already experiencing the effects of Alzheimer's. There are simple steps to the self-care necessary to prevent the decline of the brain and nervous system as a result of our daily habits.

Michael Morgan shows his deep compassion and creative genius through his work in this area. I am inspired by his book's message of hope and instructions for constructive intervention.

**Karyn M. Shanks, MD, FACP**

# TABLE OF CONTENTS

# INTRODUCTION

As a Baby Boomer growing up in the 50's and 60's, my first awareness of aging and any negative association with that process began with the word "senile." I wasn't even sure what that meant, only that it seemed to suggest some impairment of physical and mental functioning. Eventually, I heard somewhere that an accumulation of aluminum in the brain might have an influence on this disorder called "senility," which I thought about every time I consumed one of those Swanson's TV dinners, lovingly packaged in aluminum containers and wrapped in tin foil. All this before I was 15.

Decades later, the whole weight and heft of old age and mental infirmity came crashing down in front of me. I hadn't seen Edith, my stepmother, for a few years. The last I remembered, she was very warm, engaging, always polite and refined, even a bit aristocratic. Edith seemed to have always had a sense of northern Italian style. So this was my first visit to see her at the nursing home where she'd been living for some time. I went with Brenda, my stepbrother's wife. Edith was sitting on the edge of the bed. Her skin looked somehow shallow, and she had a blank stare on her face.

She looked at me for the longest time and finally said, "I know you."

"Nana, this is Michael." Brenda said.

Edith slowly turned her head to look at Brenda. After some time, she said, "I don't know you." She would continue to repeat these statements throughout the course of our visit.

I remember thinking, *What happened to Edith? Where did she go? What happened to the Edith who used to make me corn fritters and chocolate chip cookies when I came to visit her and Dad in the summer?*

We left the nursing home and I was a bit depressed. I knew Edith was there, somewhere inside, but she seemed a very long way away.

My dad, who had been dealing with this for some time, was still steadfast in his attention to her, but I could feel his anger and frustration at the situation.

Even though she hadn't yet passed away, I felt like I had already lost someone very close to me, someone who'd been an important part of my early life.

This was my introduction to Alzheimer's.

\* \* \* \* \* \* \*

Edith and my sister-in-law, Carol, both succumbed to this disease in the last few years. In Carol's case, I witnessed firsthand the gradual, and then accelerated changes in her personality and mental functioning, and watched as she began to slip away and not recognize even those closest to her. In both cases,, I eventually saw the end result of this disease, as their bodies gave out and they passed away. Of course, I not only experienced the effects of their progressive, agonizing decline and passage myself, I also saw the impact it made on their immediate families and all the caregivers, as this exhausting process took its toll.

Clearly, then, the impetus for my deep interest and involvement in studying Alzheimer's and dementia began with my family.

Fueled by all I encountered watching Edith and Carol live with and then die from Alzheimer's, I began to look at approaches that might help in the treatment of this disease, drawing on my experience and knowledge of craniosacral therapy and other natural healing modalities, to see if any of them might be of assistance. *The BodyEnergy Longevity Prescription* chronicles my journey of discovery in that pursuit—including the change of heart that arose within me, both personally and professionally, regarding "what could be done" about Alzheimer's. Indeed, my personal odyssey and years of study revealed a clear connection between the immune system and inflammation, and the factors that fuel this interaction, including diet, toxicity and lifestyle choices. In this book, we'll examine the impact on Alzheimer's of making changes in these health factors, as well as how craniosacral therapy can bring about significant positive effects to those afflicted by Alzheimer's disease and dementia.

One of the purposes in writing this book is to bring to public awareness safe, cost-effective solutions to the problems presented by Alzheimer's and dementia. My deep hope is that the current medical paradigm could become more open to alternative approaches that have shown themselves to promote significant benefit to people living with Alzheimer's—these would include craniosacral therapy, well-guided changes in diet, and other non-pharmaceutical interventions. It would also be invaluable to have the medical community partner in evaluating the effectiveness of these options.

As geriatric medicine becomes a larger part of the US medical mix and specialization, there is a tremendous opportunity to more clearly understand how seniors age, the effect of medication (or non-medication) on a more individualized, 'patient by patient' level, and further, to explore the possibility that some disease processes currently thought to be a 'one-way street' are actually treatable and perhaps even reversible. Our underlying concern in all of the above is to dramatically improve the quality of life for those who are currently healthy, those who are at risk of becoming afflicted by Alzheimer's and those who now currently challenged by the disease.

My other reason for writing *The BodyEnergy Longevity Prescription* is, not surprisingly, more personal. As a healthcare provider for over 20 years, and someone who has been impacted by the passing of two family members because of this disease, I wanted to identify a program and techniques that could easily be learned and implemented, will have no side effects, and may possibly halt or even reverse the effects of Alzheimer's and dementia. Given what I've found, observed and discovered in my quest, my greatest wish for this book is that it informs you about some truly promising possibilities, and thereby inspires you with hope.

## Chapter 1

# Our Current Dilemma

To begin, let's review the basics of the history of Alzheimer's disease and how our collective perspective about it has changed over time.

## A Brief History

The term "Alzheimer's disease" was coined in 1910 by Emil Kraepelin to acknowledge the work of German psychiatrist and neuropathologist, Alois Alzheimer, who in the early 1900's identified, diagnosed and described the disease after working with and doing a post-mortem autopsy of a patient by the name of Auguste Deter. He found it to be a progressive, degenerative disease of the brain—a form of dementia whose major symptoms are short- and long-term memory loss, confusion, mood swings, aggression, and loss of bodily functions. "Alzheimer's" was, for decades, thought to manifest in people between the ages of 45 and 65. Following a conference in 1977, the term senile dementia of the Alzheimer type (SDAT) was adopted to also describe those over 65 afflicted with such symptoms. By the 1990's the public was becoming more aware that something called Alzheimer's and/or dementia was on the rise. During that decade, over 2 million cases were reported in the US, and over 5 million worldwide.

## Current and Future Projections

Presently, Alzheimer's remains an incurable disease that has increased its reach exponentially, in terms of those it has affected. However, unlike the last few decades, when knowledge of Alzheimer's was more limited to clinical circles, today, it is a household term and commonly referred to in public discussion. This shouldn't be surprising, since in the US alone there are currently 5.4 million reported cases of Alzheimer's and more than 36 million people worldwide living with this condition. It is the 6th leading cause of death in the US, and even proportionately higher in those aged 65 and over, as one in three seniors die of dementia or related complications. It has been earmarked as a priority for research with the Obama administration, where funding is currently at 606 million dollars. And according to both a study done by the Alzheimer's Association and an article on philanthropy news source *Bloomberg,* it is recommended that research be increased twofold to $1.2 billion immediately to help counteract the spread of Alzheimer's over the next 10 years.

As for future projections, ADI's World Alzheimer's Report 2013 predicts that by 2050, Alzheimer's will effect up to 16 million seniors in the US and 115 million worldwide, reflecting a significant global health concern.

## Economic Costs

Certainly, the result of such a large increase in the number of Alzheimer's cases reaches far beyond the emotional toll it places on family, friends and caregivers (a topic I will explore more extensively in Chapter 3). The economic costs of such a dramatic rise in those afflicted by Alzheimer's needs to be addressed, as well.

Economists like to speak in terms of direct and indirect costs. For the purpose of our discussion, these can be defined as: what it costs a patient or family (direct), and what it costs the rest of society as the disease runs its course (indirect). An objective look at the current numbers involved provide insight as to why those in government, business and industry, the healthcare field and elsewhere are looking at the situation with more than a little concern. On an individual level, according to the American Alzheimer's Association's website, as of 2013, the estimated direct cost per patient is $34,500 a year with $7,259 currently coming directly out of the family's pocket (the remainder being shouldered by both governmental agencies—Medicaid, Medicare, etc.—and other social support service providers). On a national level, it's predicted that, in 2014, direct costs for Alzheimer's care in the US will be $214 billion, with indirect costs adding up to nearly $1 trillion dollars (*http://www.usagainstalzheimers.org/crisis*).

Additionally, caregivers donate or expend 17 billion hours supporting Alzheimer's-afflicted individuals, the time of which is valued at more than $216 billion annually.

Looking forward, these already massive economic costs are expected to rise substantially. According to *The World Alzheimer Report 2010: The Global Economic Impact of Dementia,* by 2030 the direct cost of Alzheimer's worldwide will grow by 85%, i.e., from the present $604 billion annual cost to over $1 trillion a year. Globally, this cost is estimated by some to be over *$20 trillion* by mid-century.

You may now be wondering how all of these facts and figures about Alzheimer's apply to the current healthcare system. Regardless of your political allegiances or opinions, you are likely aware of the concern that, over the next 10–20 years, the cost of healthcare, social security and other governmental and non-governmental costs will likely take up increasing amounts of our annual national budget, with some quite reasonably distressed that the current healthcare system may collapse. One factor contributing to this fear is that the 80–100 million Baby Boomers (those born between 1946–1965) are aging and will be reaching a stage where they will be in need of services over the next few decades. Certainly, not all of these healthcare system concerns are related to Alzheimer's and dementia. Still, with an aging population on the rise, an increasing percentage of these national budgets can significantly (and relatively quickly) consume resources.

I believe, however, there is some good news in the face of this pressing, widespread and highly challenging health issue. The urgency and growing concern about our ability to cover ever-increasing healthcare costs inadvertently creates an opportunity to look at alternative approaches. This is especially notable if such approaches are preventative in nature, cost-effective, or cost-neutral relative to existing avenues, and evidence-based in their approach.

## The Current Senior Care System

### Alzheimer's, Diabetes, and Heart Disease
### Quick Facts for US Population

#### Alzheimer's:
- Projected 115.4 million worldwide by 2050
- Sixth leading cause of death
- 1 in 3 seniors die with Dementia or related complications
- 5.4 million currently diagnosed

#### Diabetes
- 28.5 million children and adults.
- Another 7 million undiagnosed, or more than 10% of the population
- On the rise in the younger population and expected to increase.
- 1 in 3 adults in the US could have diabetes by 2050
- 79 million (20 or over are estimated to have Pre-diabetes.
- In ages 65 or older, 26.9% of the population are diagnosed
- Seventh leading cause of death

#### Heart Disease
- 26.5 million non-institutionalized adults or 6% of the population
- Number one cause of death

There are a few more facts and figures to discuss in order to round out the picture of how our present healthcare system is caring for those afflicted by Alzheimer's. First, we'll briefly review how professionals in the medical field are treating patients living with Alzheimer's disease and dementia. Then, we will touch on the approaches and practices being used in many nursing homes and other assisted living institutions that offer long-term care for Alzheimer's patients, as well as the support and challenges that at-home caregivers and families are facing.

"Quality of life" is a term often heard in the senior care industry, and we will look at that, as well.

## Current Approaches

Given there is a great deal of research being conducted on Alzheimer's, which I will review in the following chapter, let's take a quick overview of our existing approaches to treating the disease, including current medical and institutional practices. As was mentioned earlier, there is no known cure for Alzheimer's. The best approach, at the moment, is to, at the very least, delay the onset of the disease. This has resulted in the use of such medications as Aricept and the Exelon patch. The results of the administration of such drugs has had mixed results, but offers a resource to those in need of assistance. As Alzheimer's progresses and brain tissue degenerates, both of these drugs seem to be less effective.

Not surprisingly, researchers have come to realize over the years that since the effects of the disease in the advanced stages is so devastating, it makes sense to both study, and if possible, treat the disease at an earlier stage. This has resulted in a growing awareness of the importance of identifying early symptoms and has brought into usage such terms as mild cognitive impairment (MCI), in an attempt to describe and also treat potential onset of Alzheimer's at an earlier stage. Unfortunately, options for early intervention and treatment—with the exception of the medical interventions mentioned above—are still basically nonexistent. That is, in part, the reason why the BodyEnergy Longevity Prescription emerged as a response: *we are taking a different view of the disease process and providing an intervention that offers additional options.*

While almost everyone agrees that early identification and treatment is critical, it is a matter of debate as to what measures may be the most effective in slowing or stopping the progression of the disease. As an adjunct to current research, the identification of genetic markers has received a good deal of attention, which may give us some indication of who may develop the disease in later years. In general, the genetic approach has become a popular way to look at disease processes, as genetic engineering offers a long-term promise in the treatment of a wide variety of diseases.

Our current methods of treating Alzheimer's also reflect how families have approached caring for those in their midst who are living with this condition. As I recounted earlier in my experience with my stepmother Edith and my sister-in-law, Carol, because of Alzheimer's' direct impact on memory and cognition, it is as if those closest to us begin to slip away. In a very real sense, it is like losing someone before they pass on. The particular issues involved in living with this "loss" also bring about a specific need for support and understanding. Resources like the American Alzheimer's Association (*www.alz.org*), Alzheimer's Foundation of America (*http://alzfdn.org/*) and Maria Shriver (*www.alz.org/mariashriver*) offer various support structures for families and caregivers.

Presently, the way we care for our loved ones afflicted with Alzheimer's is often reflected in the kind of senior living community we employ to serve them. As was mentioned earlier, such facilities are equipped with various resources, among them assisted living staff and skilled nursing, with some featuring specialized memory units. In addition to the options provided by senior living communities and nursing homes, a family's economics and preferences can also make at-home-care the avenue taken to support the family member living with Alzheimer's. Certainly, living with family impacts both the support of an Alzheimer's patient and the family members themselves. A recent study points to caregiving as a leading stressor for families, with more than half (52.8%) of those caring for individuals with diseases such as cancer and Alzheimer's presenting scores indicating depression.

As our population ages and the economy changes, the mix of in-home and institutionalized care may change as well—more seniors being cared for by family members, for example—and this will be reflected in the stresses that caregivers face, much like the challenges other groups face, such as those raising children with special needs.

## My Story Begins

Early in 2006, I began to think about how craniosacral therapy might impact the treatment of Alzheimer's and dementia, based on Dr. John E. Upledger's comments about the flow of cerebral spinal fluid (CSF) in individuals as they age. I brought this idea to one of my clients, a researcher at the University of Iowa, and out of this initial idea emerged a proposal to study Alzheimer's and dementia with some simple craniosacral techniques. Dr. Upledger was supportive of this proposal, and over time there emerged a study that was published in the Volume 34 (2008) issue of the *Journal of Gerontological Nursing* ("CranioSacral StillPoint Technique: Exploring Its Effects in Individuals with Dementia," Gerdner, et al). I acted as a consultant on the craniosacral therapy aspect of the study and created the teams of therapists who administered it, both in Iowa and Minnesota.[1]

In a very real sense, this was a starting point for my conducting further investigation. As is often the case, information can come to us in unexpected ways. Sometime after the study was published, I was speaking with a gentleman who was on the board of directors of the Southern California Alzheimer's Association. He said to me, "You know, Mike, about 40% of people in an Alzheimer's unit have diabetes." Well, no, I didn't know that. And it sparked a curiosity in me. After all, 40% is a fairly significant figure. Since I often find in the craniosacral therapy classes I teach people who work in nursing home environments, I decided to informally ask them if they noticed a significant number of Alzheimer's patients with diabetes. Though this was not a rigorous scientific way of gathering data, I did find their responses often confirmed these figures.

## Connecting Ideas

The plot, as they say, began to thicken. As I started to think about the connection between diabetes and Alzheimer's, I also began to go back and look at Dr. Upledger's comments about Alzheimer's and dementia. Dr. Upledger, who is brilliant generally, but especially in the area of biochemistry, had created a series of classes based on his lifetime

[1] more on the background to the study can be found in chapter 6

of observing the human immune system. As an aspect of this, he also looked at the potential to reverse the pathogenic process. Central to his observation was the role of inflammation in creating disease processes, with Alzheimer's being one of them. So, I began to look at the details of his observations, and was able to use them to supplement my own thoughts about how craniosacral therapy could both augment and add to current studies and research on the subject.

My research continued, and I began to realize that many people who display symptoms of Alzheimer's and dementia have a history of prior disease processes—some existing over decades—before this particular disease shows noticeable signs. I also found that, according to the American Autoimmune Related Diseases Association, numerous studies have indicated that many of these dysfunctions may have been caused by inflammation, among them arthritis, osteoporosis, diabetes, cardiac disease, cancer, and depression. This is not to say that everyone with these symptoms will develop Alzheimer's, but there are some links that bear further investigation.

I am not the first one to arrive at some of these same conclusions. In addition to Dr. Upledger's contribution, I would also like to acknowledge a number of thinkers and researchers who are ahead of their time: Dr. Andrew Weil, who pioneered valuable concepts that helped train and retrain medical professionals in holistic medicine; Dr. Jeffrey Bland, considered by many to be "the father of functional medicine;" Dr. Mark Hyman, who has played a huge role in bringing inflammatory disease and the epidemic of diabetes into national focus; and Dr. Dean Ornish, who with his pioneering research, introduced the concept that a disease process such as cardiovascular disease is not just treatable, but actually reversible. I will touch more on each one of these researchers, as the story in this book unfolds. There are many others I could name, but these particular gentlemen deserve special mention. Of course, in this list, I must also mention my own functional medicine specialist, Dr. Karyn Shanks, who has taught me personally that both recovery and healing after decades of abuse and neglect are possible.

## What We Are Presenting—The Whole vs. the Parts

Early on when I began my craniosacral practice, I needed a name for my new company. It seemed obvious that the changes I saw in my clients were reflected in positive and increased energy in their bodies; hence, the BodyEnergy Company was born. As my research and observations about craniosacral therapy, diet, inflammation and other supporting modalities began to take shape, the concept of a 'BodyEnergy Longevity Prescription' emerged. This approach, as you'll see, unwaveringly aims to address the "whole" picture of what's going on with Alzheimer's disease.

Given that inflammation has been linked to the onset of many disease processes, it seemed important to me to examine whether or not inflammation could be a contributing factor to Alzheimer's disease, and if so, how cranialsacral therapy, my own specialty, could have the ability to make a positive effect in its treatment One key component of craniosacral therapy is to look at the whole person and appreciate how each piece of information from a patient's body forms a mosaic or pattern. What we teach our students in this therapy is to go beyond identifying symptoms and to look for the generator or cause of the problem. When studying the history of Alzheimer's, it makes sense to look at what osteopaths call the "lesional chain" or connection from one incident or trauma to another. My experience has been that when we look at the history of a person with Alzheimer's, we often discover that the symptom of Alzheimer's is the tip of the iceberg. In digging beneath the surface, we find that numerous instances of prior inflammatory processes in the brain precede the identification of Alzheimer's, often by decades.

To uncover what's really taking place, I began following the evidence, starting with an examination of the current research in the field. I was especially aware of the importance of using my expertise as a craniosacral therapist in listening to the processes of the body, including the flow of cerebral spinal fluid, to detect the existence of inflammation and whether or not it could have an influence in the formation of the disease.

As we proceed forward, then, I will show how inflammation and the way it is moderated by the immune system begins in the body and eventually, in some cases, overflows into the brain, creating the symptoms of Alzheimer's and dementia. I will weave into this story the concepts of craniosacral therapy, which give us a different perspective on how to prevent, arrest and even reverse the effect of the disease.

The starting point in my inquiry was Dr. Upledger's observations on the relationship between the immune system and inflammation. He noted that inflammation is a response of the body and specifically, the immune system. The brain responds to the immune system's mobilization as a sort of overreaction to a specific stimuli (just like when one sprains an ankle, the foot swells up) and increases its response to the problem as it deems necessary, resulting in varying degrees of inflammation. I refer to these stages of inflammation as the Brain-Inflammatory Response.

From here, the trail of breadcrumbs—from an inflammatory point of view—went "backwards," in that I began examining how other inflammatory conditions can accumulate in the body and account for a wide variety of maladies that we often see at various stages in our lives. What I found was that many of these maladies also involve the immune system. Typically, the standard medical model approaches these challenges from a pharmaceutical point of view, which often ends up suppressing the immune system *and* the inflammatory response in order to achieve a desired effect. *The BodyEnergy Longevity Prescription* (which includes craniosacral therapy) utilizes more natural processes to moderate this response. With this approach, we are actually using the inner wisdom of the body to find other ways to respond to the challenges that can create long-term problems.

Eventually, at "the end of the trail," I saw the importance of taking into account the relationship between the foods we eat and how the immune system may react to them over time. Researchers such as Dr. Mark Hyman, who coined the term "diabesity," clearly pointed out the relationship between weight gain and insulin resistance, elaborating with further details about "metabolic syndrome" and other mechanisms that help explain the importance of what we consume and how it affects our body.

## Reversal is Possible

It is at this point in my quest that I realized craniosacral therapy and other modalities began to complement each other and, when used together in a coordinated treatment protocol, offer a profound and exciting possibility for those living with Alzheimer's disease.

In Chapter 11, based on the initial observations of a pilot study discussed in a 2008 edition of the *American Journal of Geriatric Nursing* mentioned above ("Reversal of Alzheimer's and Dementia—A Bold Proposal"), I present a model or hypothesis for how Alzheimer's can be prevented, arrested and even reversed in terms of the damage caused to the brain. To better convey this hypothetical approach for addressing Alzheimer's, I use the analogy of putting out a forest fire, obviously to illustrate inflammation as a sort of fire in the brain. In the model, I discuss three stages of treatment for contending with Alzheimer's. The first stage, *Containing the Blaze,* proposes the use of craniosacral therapy (CST) to help increase cerebrospinal fluid flow to the brain and help decrease or diminish inflammation. The second stage, *Extinguishing the Fire,* continues to utilize daily applications of CST and boldly proposes an institutional change in diet and nutrition with the thinking that an anti-inflammatory diet, as proposed by functional medicine doctors and others, will help reduce the "dry tinder" in the metabolic processes of the body that keeps fueling the inflammation. Finally, in Stage 3, *Reseeding the Forest,* we continue with practices outlined in the first two stages and add other techniques from advanced CST that could help repair nerve and brain tissue damage. Here, I also reference literature from others, including Dr. Dean Ornish, to illustrate how repair of this type is possible.

## What Is at Stake and the Possibility of Cultural Change

I had no idea when I started looking at the connection between Alzheimer's and dementia, craniosacral therapy and quality of life that I would discover a silent, but growing national health crisis. However, that is exactly what I found! Let me share some statistics and let you draw your own conclusions. There are currently 25 million people in the US diagnosed with diabetes with another estimated 7 million who are undiagnosed. There are an estimated 79 million people who are pre-diabetic. Add all these people together and you get over 100 million people, or about one-third of the US population, who are or will be affected by diabetes. Further, it is estimated that in 20 years, one in two people will be diabetic or pre-diabetic. When you factor time and age into this combination, a certain percentage of those people will develop cardiovascular disease, as well, and a certain percentage of those will develop dementia or Alzheimer's. Of course, not all of these factors are clearly linked, *but there is a relationship between them.* Now, what we don't know yet is the exact percentage. It could be 2%, 10% or 20%, or higher! Regardless of the exact percentage, Alzheimer's has been described as the defining disease of the Baby Boomer generation (Maria Shriver, "Alzheimer's: A Baby Boomer Epidemic" May 8, 2009, *Huffington Post*).

What I am doing is attempting to show a viable connection between Alzheimer's, inflammation, diet and life-style. Fortunately, others such as Dr. Mark Hyman and Dr. William Davis have laid the groundwork, explaining how the inflammatory nature of some foods creates insulin resistance, diabetes and obesity. Others, such as Dr. Dean Ornish, have documented how diet and cardiovascular disease are linked. When you look at the actual direct and indirect costs (summed together to include the direct costs to families and the government, and the indirect cost to business and industry, and each and every one of us), the estimated *total* cost to the US economy by the year 2050 varies anywhere from 1.2 trillion to 20 trillion dollars. The loss of creativity and energy cannot truly be factored into this equation.

These astronomical figures naturally lead one to ask, "Who is going to pay this bill?" With over 80 million Baby Boomers on the verge of retirement (if they can afford to), will it not be the younger generations who'll be forced to bear the burden of this ongoing support?

Some people have described the current US healthcare system as broken, while others describe it as a "sick care" system. Many see it as a system that "rewards" disease and reimburses countless medical providers for treatment with a focus on reducing symptoms, *regardless* of whether this is the best or healthiest approach. Quite frankly, it's obvious there is no magic pill (no pun intended) that will cure the problems entrenching our healthcare system.

As for addressing Alzheimer's, I sincerely hope that a particular pharmaceutical treatment *will* be developed that counteracts this devastating disease. However, the evidence suggests that the underlying causes are complex and must be addressed at a more fundamental level, a fact which is reflected in a variety of other diseases across the entire spectrum of the population. Of course, the traditional approaches can still be employed. My only question is, "Can the US economy continue to afford the end effect of supporting lifestyles that promote the inflammatory response and the resulting related diseases with a focus on treating symptoms only, while ignoring the underlying causes?"

It seems obvious that the issues facing our healthcare system, especially those related to Alzheimer's and dementia, are not going to be resolved overnight. In the interim, there are other approaches that can be of assistance. Craniosacral therapy is simple, efficient and has no side effects. It is also easily administered and non-invasive. It is a manual, motion producing therapy, and motion is essential to maintaining health and vibrancy in the body. The reason we need CST in addition to dietary and lifestyle changes is that once the inflammatory process has progressed, those afflicted with Alzheimer's need additional assistance to quell the inflammation. The fire needs to be controlled, and if possible, extinguished, and then the fuel feeding the fire removed.

There is one last point we need to consider when addressing the differences between traditional medical treatments for Alzheimer's and therapies such as CST. If we compare the ongoing healthcare costs of treating just the symptoms and the resulting degeneration, to the support costs for CST administration and training, the cost for the latter are *minimal.* It is this type of approach that will become even more attractive as economic pressures increase. Oh yes, let's not forget improvement in quality of life for those living with Alzheimer's, which *really* should be at the top of our list.

## Join the Adventure

I invite you to read through the remaining chapters of this book and share in the journey I've been on over the last few years. Hopefully, you too will see how all these factors interconnect, as you look at how much progress has been made by brilliant researchers who have been earnestly searching for a cure; as you read through some of the personal stories of caregivers; as you review Dr. Upledger's unique contribution of craniosacral therapy; and as you examine the research done connecting CST and Alzheimer's. Continuing forward, you'll see how inflammation, the immune system and the brain interact, and what contributes to this inflammation. In addition, you will be shown some of the obstacles to changing how we think, and then how the momentum of aging can be addressed, even after the accumulation of stress and strain. Finally, I will invite you to become part of this adventure, and help create a new vision for an integrated healthcare plan for ourselves, our seniors and all future generations to come.

## Chapter 2

# History and Current Research

In this chapter, we will take a more in-depth look at Alzheimer's, its current medical description, and the presumed cause of this disease. As part of this examination, we will look at the current models to explain the mechanism of Alzheimer's and what the top researchers in the field have to say. I will also use this as a counterpoint to my research and compare and contrast it with the BodyEnergy and craniosacral therapy approach.

## The Origin of "Alzheimer's"

Alois Alzheimer, a psychiatrist, began working with a patient in 1902 who displayed signs of dementia. He tracked the progression of her symptoms (loss of memory, confusion, irritability, delusions, aggression, even temporary vegetative states) through 1906, at which time he reported his findings. He was the first to identify the disease's primary symptoms of loss of memory and cognitive abilities over time. Very early on, researchers began to call this dysfunction Alzheimer's disease, with a number of cases being tracked and reported through the next few decades. In 1977, a conference on Alzheimer's disease concluded that the symptoms of pre-senile and senile dementia were almost the same, and the more official terminology of senile dementia of the Alzheimer type (SDAT) was adopted to describe the condition in those over 65. Over time, the medical nomenclature adapted these official terms and descriptions.

### "What is the Cause?"—Current Theories Point to Brain Plaques and Tangles

There are a number of theories as to what causes Alzheimer's, but most of them agree that the evidence of moderate to severe Alzheimer's is reflected in plaques and neurofibrillary tangles found in the brain. These plaques and tangles, typically discovered during autopsies of those who have passed away from the disease, are extremely destructive to brain tissue and seem to be the cause of loss of memory and cognitive function. What is unknown is exactly how the plaques and tangles are formed. Most researchers agree that part of the mechanism of their formation comes from amyloid precursor proteins (APP's) that are broken down, as evidenced by the existence of enzymes or secretases called beta, gamma and tau proteins, which cut the APP into fragments. Those, in turn, become the plaques and tangles embedded in the brain.

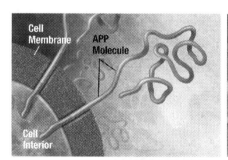

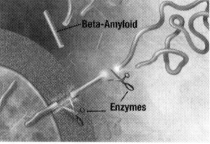

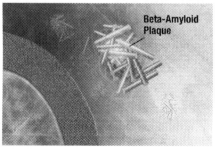

What follows is a summary of what the leading researchers in Alzheimer's have to say, and a reflection about research in the field in general. I will also offer some comments about how these perspectives may counter or support my findings, as I developed the BodyEnergy Longevity Prescription. Then, we'll look at the history of the BodyEnergy Longevity Prescription, and the evidence and information that supports this "downstream" approach.

Now, before proceeding, you may be asking, "What does 'downstream approach' mean?" One of the terms researchers use is "downstream," meaning they believe there is a cascade of events that precede the actual formation of plaques and tangles. This is a good news/bad news scenario. The good news is that by looking at a series of events that precede the actual event, it acknowledges a series of complex interactions that lead to a final result. Nature is, as we know, sometimes fickle. In the case of Alzheimer's and other diseases, the inner intelligence of the body and brain will react in a variety of ways to a perceived threat from the outside. These 'downstream events,' depending on how far back we go, could include the influence of such things as exposure to toxins, unhealthy foods and metals, or just the inherent reaction of the body trying to maintain equilibrium. I support the downstream concept and, indeed, the BodyEnergy Prescription takes into account events that typically precede the formation of Alzheimer's and dementia by decades.

The bad news about looking downstream, from a scientific point of view, is that the further back in time one goes, whether it be seconds, minutes, days or years, it is harder to quantify or control the variables. This means that the understanding of the causal mechanism is less precise, from a researcher's point of view. However, the BodyEnergy Prescription's approach is more practical. If the factors discussed in this book are taken into account, we may be able to come up with a solution that will prevent the incidence of Alzheimer's in the first place. And, in those cases where the disease already exists, we may be able to stop and even reverse the progression of the disease.

## Current Research

As one may surmise from the above, 'downstream researchers' acknowledge the accumulation of factors from the past and their importance. John C. Morris, MD, Professor of Neurology, Pathology & Immunology, Physical Therapy, and Occupational Therapy at Washington University in St. Louis, is a pioneering downstream researcher. In a Science Watch interview with correspondent Gary Taubes (Oct. 2011), he gives his perspective of the formation of Alzheimer's:

*"How do you think researchers have to approach Alzheimer's disease to make the most progress? And how has this philosophy driven your own research?*

> *"At the risk of being over-simplistic, here's what I think: the Alzheimer's disease process occurs over many years, perhaps decades. The earliest stages of the disease begin with dysregulation of the amyloid-beta protein, such that it is overproduced or under-cleared (or both). These abnormalities eventually result in the cerebral deposition of amyloid plaques and ultimately are marked by a cascade of pathological events that culminate in neurodegeneration.*
>
> *"This process may take place over many years in the absence of any detectable symptoms. Ultimately the accumulating pathologies reach a threshold where the integrity of neurons is compromised, and you begin to get dysfunction and ultimately death. When there is sufficient dysfunction of synapses and neurons, then brain function is impaired and the symptoms of Alzheimer's disease gradually become apparent."*

Professor Morris' summary, which he cautions may be somewhat over-simplistic, bears out my experience. I have observed in my own practice that, based on palpation or 'listening' to the craniosacral rhythm (which reflects the pumping action of cerebralspinal fluid), it is fairly easy to feel restrictions in the membrane system of a senior's cranium. These restrictions become more noticeable, as a patient progresses from 'at risk' to early onset to mid stage Alzheimer's and beyond. In addition, such restrictions are often accompanied by a sense of inflammation in the cranium, which most advanced CST practitioners can

# Alzheimer's Disease: A Molecular Misstep?
# The Current Research Model

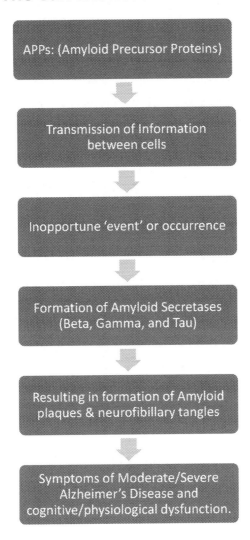

also sense. In other words, from a craniosacral point of view, evidence exists to show the physiological and structural interference or restrictions in the brain that results in what Dr. Morris deems 'under cleared' production of amyloid-beta protein. It is also likely that greater inflammation in the central nervous system, caused by these restrictions, is a contributing factor to an overproduction of amyloid-beta protein. Our point is that, through simple CST palpation, it is possible to detect the beginning of this process in advance of a formal diagnosis.

Another researcher, Dr. Jeffrey Cummings, MD, Director of Cleveland Clinic's Lou Ruvo Center for Brain Health (in Las Vegas) and Professor of Neurotherapeutics and Drug Development for the Cleveland Clinic's Neurological Institute, provides a slightly different perspective:

> *"The field in general is moving toward earlier and earlier diagnosis. We've realized that by the time the patient reaches the current criteria for dementia, there is very substantial brain injury present. For our drugs to work and to preserve the patients' function at the highest possible level, we need to diagnose them at earlier phases in the disease.*
>
> *"That's why there's so much emphasis on mild cognitive impairment and what's called prodromal Alzheimer's disease. This means the patient does not meet the clinical criteria for Alzheimer's dementia, which is how we currently diagnose Alzheimer's disease, but we believe the disease is already present in the brain. Then the question is, how do we show that?"*

Professor Cummings points out, here, the importance of early identification, which is an observation heralded by many researchers. After all, researchers have found that the earlier the disease is identified, the less damage there is to the brain. (This push for earlier identification actually helped Alzheimer's specialists identify what is termed "mild cognitive impairment" or MCI.) Professor Cummings and others seem to have a keen eye focused on whatever may be capable of arresting the progression of the disease. The BodyEnergy approach, which offers just such a possibility, will be more thoroughly discussed in later chapters.

In addition to Professors Morris and Cummings, there are some researchers who echo the importance of the amyloid beta peptide or enzyme in the formation of plaques and tangles. In 2011, Dr. Mark Mattson of the National Institute of Aging, stated:

> *"Bruce Yankner at Harvard was the first to show that the amyloid beta peptide can damage and kill neurons, and we followed*

*up closely on his findings and started to elucidate the molecular
mechanism responsible for the damaging effects of this peptide.*

*"We found two main processes going on. One was that this pep-
tide, when it's self-aggregating, causes oxidative stress, and this
seems to be particularly bad when the peptide is aggregating
on the surface of nerve cells. We showed that the oxidative stress
caused by amyloid disrupts calcium regulation in the neurons and
makes them very vulnerable to, for example, the damaging effects
of glutamate receptor activation or to reduced energy levels.*

*"Some think that during normal aging, the ability of nerve
cells to maintain energy levels is reduced. So if amyloid is accu-
mulating along with the changes induced by normal aging, the
amyloid might tip the neurons over the edge and cause them to
degenerate."*

Clearly, Professor Mattson's comments indicate the possible cumulative effect and damage of the amyloid beta peptide on nerve and
brain tissue.

Dr. Denis Selkoe, Professor of Neurologic Diseases at Harvard,
shares this point of view from a slightly different perspective, emphasizing molecular imbalance as a key factor:

*"My opinion is that there is an imbalance between the produc-
tion and the removal of a small hydrophobic protein called amyloid
beta that triggers the process we call Alzheimer's. I believe that
imbalance arises from a lot of different, more fundamental causes.
What I'm saying is that amyloid beta is both necessary and, at
least in some cases, sufficient to cause Alzheimer's disease, but
there are many other factors."*

He goes on to suggest the best path forward for treating
Alzheimer's:

*"If we had to choose one, and I think the clearest, path to treat-
ment, it would be targeting amyloid beta, rather than any of these
other factors, including tau, which looks like it comes downstream
in the Alzheimer's cascade. So to summarize, my opinion is that it's
an imbalance of amyloid beta protein in the brain that triggers or
precipitates Alzheimer's."*

However there are some dissenting opinions, as well. Dr. George Perry, Dean of the College of Sciences at the University of Texas in San Antonio, suggests the opposite of the amyloid beta theory:

> *"Ours is that amyloid is a response to the disease, not the cause of the disease. Amyloid is not irrelevant. It's very, very important.*
>
> *"Why? There are several reasons. One is vaccines. When amyloid is removed from brains using vaccines, it doesn't help patients. In fact, patients got slightly worse. This is true in all the studies. Further, when one sees amyloid deposition in the brain, oxidative damage decreases. So there's an inverse correlation. Whether oligomers or fibers, when we see amyloid increased, we see a decrease in the levels of oxidative damage. One important mechanism for amyloid's apparent antioxidant activity is that it binds copper and redox silences it.*
>
> *"With my colleague Mark A. Smith, also a highly cited person who unfortunately died in December, we've written probably about 100 publications questioning the amyloid-cascade hypothesis.*
>
> *"The amyloid cascade hypothesis is a very simplistic view that was useful to consolidate many observations under testable hypotheses. Failure of those tests has now put the hypothesis in question. Unfortunately, the cascade hypothesis is fundamentally a biological concept. It goes against evolutionary selection; it does so by proposing a well-adjusted organism would produce a response that has but a detrimental effect. For a response to develop in the body, it must have some adaptive value."*

Dr. Perry's comments above reflect the current uncertainty in understanding of exactly how nature works. The concept of "who is the culprit" is active here, and I think sparks healthy dialogue. I must make note that my mentor, Dr. John Upledger, made somewhat of the same observations years ago. He noted that amyloid exists in the body with no ill effect and, indeed, seems to have a positive effect or at the very least can coexist with other body systems. So the concept of amyloid being a response to the disease, rather than the cause, is a valuable one. Later, I will be discussing the role of the immune system and inflammatory processes in the body and brain, and there I will note that these reflect Dr. Perry's observations, as well.

In an October 2011 Science Watch interview, Dr. David Bennett, Professor of Neurological Sciences & Director of the Rush Alzheimer's Disease Center at Rush Medial College in Chicago, discussed the nature of disappointment in Alzheimer's (drug) trials:

**Science Watch:** *Why do you think that is (that drug trials have not been conclusive)?*

*"For a variety of reasons. First, a lot of the drugs we tried don't work because we really don't know enough about the basic biology of what's going on in Alzheimer's. Sometimes we're trying things with a hope and a prayer. And then, where the biology is worked out well—say, with the amyloid modulators—a lot of us think that we're giving them too late in the disease process and that interfering with amyloid metabolism probably needs to be done way before people have dementia, possibly before they have mild cognitive impairment.*

*"Unfortunately, we don't know how to do prevention trials in a cost-effective way. When you try to figure out what it would take, they become hugely expensive. This is one of the factors driving biomarkers studies. The thought is that if you can follow a biomarker, rather than following the clinical course itself, you can do these studies with a smaller sample size and a shorter duration.*

*"A good example is in HIV research. Researchers used to take people who were HIV positive and wait for them to get AIDS. When they started using CD4 counts as a proxy, the sample sizes came down, the duration of the studies came down, and the costs came down. The speed with which they could work their way through various agents markedly increased. It would be great if we could find something like that for Alzheimer's disease. So far, we have found some markers, but not markers that could be used as surrogate outcomes in clinical trials."*

I think Dr. Bennett's comments are an honest reflection of the trial and error nature of research. It may seem a bit harsh, but he points out that the smaller the sample and the later the progression of the disease, the easier, in a sense, it is to study. What this means, practically speaking, is that the best way to study this population is to wait until they are far past the point of no return, in terms of clinical intervention. Only those who are most certainly terminal will give a better predictable outcome. However, this approach can only end up being "good for the study, bad for the patient."

There are a few more points we would do well to consider. Since the impact of genetics has become so popular in recent years, I thought I would include another statement by Dr. Bennett regarding genetic risk factors:

> "One is that a variety of genetic factors associated with the clinical diagnosis of Alzheimer's disease seem to be related to the typical pathologies we think of as causing the disease, which is amyloid deposition and neurofibrillary tangle formation. Traditionally, Alzheimer's is somebody with cognitive decline, dementia, and these two pathologies in the brain at death. We generally think that risk factors for Alzheimer's dementia as causing this pathology.
>
> "That's true for genetic risk factors. It turns out that when we get to experiential risk factors, such as cognitive activity, physical activity, social activity, education, and psychological factors that also predict clinical Alzheimer's disease, such as depression, neuroticism, conscientiousness, loneliness, and harm avoidance, and we've reported a large number of these factors related to cognitive decline and getting clinical Alzheimer's, none of these seem to be causing amyloid deposition or tangle formation. None of them."

In later chapters, I will discuss epigenetics, or the study of changes in gene expressions that have other causes than changes in the DNA sequence—which includes the theory that genes can be switched on or off to support healthy functioning in the body and brain. Epigenetics arose, at least in part, from the observation that some people who have a very similar background and history could show signs of a disease, but not display any definitive negative signs of it.

I make mention of epigenetics at this point, because there has been some lively discussion about genetics and its role in Alzheimer's and dementia. Since there is currently no known cure for Alzheimer's, even if genetic markers for the disease were identified, many people simply may not want to know. However, *The BodyEnergy Longevity Prescription* offers a new point of view: that by careful listening to the body, and soliciting advice from the inner wisdom of a patient, it may be possible to help 'turn off' the genetic factors that are detrimental to brain functioning, while at the same time 'switch on' genetic expressions that may be more favorable to a patient's overall health and mental well-being. This would be, in essence, the fulfillment of the approach epigenetics takes.

Finally, let's look at a few more comments from Dr. Cummings, drawn from his being interviewed about the newest field of amyloid scans, made possible by a company that has developed a radioactive tracer that allows beta amyloid to be imaged by sophisticated technology:

> *"This is a year of great excitement for us, because it looks like an amyloid-imaging scan is likely to be approved by the FDA for widespread use. This is essentially a diagnostic test for Alzheimer's disease. And it's a game-changer in terms of identifying patients and allowing us to develop more specific patient populations for intervention studies."*

**Science Watch:** *Can you quantify how accurate this is at establishing the presence of amyloid in subject's brains?*

> *"Well, we believe it's very accurate. Almost every patient with Alzheimer's disease will have amyloid visible on this scan. Patients in the mild cognitive impairment phase who have Alzheimer's disease as a cause of their mild cognitive impairment also have positive scans. So the scan has high predictive value for saying which patients with mild cognitive impairment are going to progress to Alzheimer's-type dementia."*

Now again, this is a mixture of good news and bad news. Meaning, given that a possible test for Alzheimer's has been developed, there will certainly be individuals who would not want to have the diagnosis, especially if there is not currently a cure. However, from the BodyEnergy point of view, a natural curiosity arises. This is because long-term studies could examine moderate to severe Alzheimer's patients and, utilizing these radioactive tracers do scans of patients before and after the application of craniosacral techniques. This technology provides us with the potential, here, to show in this imaging the direct effect of this "hands on" technique.

# Alzheimer's Disease: A Molecular Misstep? The BodyEnergy View

Inflammatory Response (May have existed for years or decades e.g. diabetes, heart disease, arthritis

Proinflammatory Cytokines overflow into the brain

Proinflammatory Response cause acute phase response in brain (e.g. more inflammation, memory loss. lethargy)

APPs (amyloid precursor proteins) transmission of information between cells.

Formation of Amyloid Secretases (Beta, Gamma, and Tau)

Resulting in formation of Amyloid plaques & neurofibillary tangles

Symptoms of Moderate/Severe Alzheimer's Disease and cognitive/physiological dysfunction.

To summarize, this overview of current research on Alzheimer's disease demonstrates:

- There are many dedicated scientists looking for a way to explain the causes and effects of Alzheimer's. Most of them would agree that "the smoking gun" has something to do with the amyloid beta peptides, which seem to be in evidence when plaques and tangles in the brain are formed.
- A number of current theories diverge, when it comes to precisely describing what exactly causes what.

In the next chapter, we will put a human face on the impact of Alzheimer's and dementia, and look at the very real impact it has on our families, friends and countless people in every community throughout the world.

## Chapter 3

# A Family Affair Memoirs, Inspiration and Hope

During my research into Alzheimer's and dementia, I inevitably found the American Alzheimer's Association's website, which led me also to sites for the inspiring work being done by Maria Shriver and Leeza Gibbons. As I examined these sites and recalled my own personal experiences, I saw there are literally thousands of accounts of those impacted by the onset of this disease. (In the U.S., it turns out to be 1 in 6!) I felt somewhat like Jim Carrey's character in the film, *Bruce Almighty,* when he was able to hear the prayers of everyone all at the same time. While I am not claiming any divine abilities, I sensed all of these people were crying out for answers. I thought, *If they're given a reason to feel hopeful, and an effective, non-toxic treatment protocol, that could radiate positively to countless others in their lives, potentially improving the lives of millions of people.*

As I followed through with this line of thinking, I naturally began to see what a profound effect craniosacral therapy might have when given to Alzheimer's patients (especially when combined with a number of other health measures). The following account provides some sense of what is possible when CST is applied, showing the effect on both patients and caregivers.

## A Lesson From Russia

One of my first revelations about the potentially huge positive impact CST could have on people with Alzheimer's and their families came from a most unlikely place: Moscow, Russia. I was teaching a class I'd developed entitled, "CranioSacral Therapy for Longevity: Reversal of the Aging Process," to a group of particularly talented osteopaths and healthcare professionals from all over that vast nation. We require volunteers to come in to the class, so the students can apply the new techniques they've just learned. One of our senior volunteers was accompanied by her daughter and son-in-law. Even with no Russian language skills at all, it was clear to me, by the look on the daughter's face, that she was very concerned about her mother.

The doctor proceeded to practice his newly learned hands-on skills, assisted by another health professional, applying the treatment process to the mother. The most amazing thing about the treatment session was not the look on her face, or her ability to recognize others, or even the perceivable difference in her walking gait and flexibility, all of which changed for the better in 30 minutes. No, it was the *clearly noticeable* change in her relationship with her daughter that stood out to me (and likely to all who were witnessing this session). I found out that the daughter and mother had been somewhat estranged and out of communication for several years, even choosing to live in different parts of Russia. Only recently, because of the mother's illness, had the daughter come to visit. What was surprising was that after this one initial session, both mom and daughter spent half the night talking with each other and reconnecting in a most profound way.

I am convinced the CST treatment opened the pathway for increased cognition on the part of the mother and also gave the daughter hope, as she realized she had access to her mother in ways she felt would never have been possible again. So encouraged was this family, they insisted on coming back again the next day. This time, they came with the husband, the daughter, the son-in-law and two grandchildren, including a totally charming 4-year-old. All three generations participated in the treatment, literally linked together for 45 minutes, with the 4-year-old seemingly directing the whole affair from the feet of her grandmother. It was as if a multigenerational family history was acknowledged, changed and shifted in this process. Also, the student/doctor was able to show the daughter some of the simple CST techniques and recommend that she administer them to her mother on a daily basis, which is part of the BodyEnergy Longevity Prescription I'll soon be discussing more fully.

As I recalled the following cases of people with Alzheimer's (some who I knew personally and others not) and the effects levied on the respective families, I looked forward into the future and wondered just how significant it would be if CST were adopted worldwide as a supportive treatment protocol for people with Alzheimer's, if it could make such a difference—as it had with that Russian mother and her daughter—in patients' and families' lives all over the world.

The following stories are further examples of the personal impact that Alzheimer's has had on the family, and they also demonstrate the progression of the disease—from early signs, to "things going downhill," and ultimately, to the end of life.


## Ronald Reagan

Many people are familiar with the plight of former President Ronald Reagan and his struggle with Alzheimer's. Although I was much younger at the time, I remember the speech he gave, a farewell in a sense, after he learned of his diagnosis and pending journey into this unknown area. This was a very public sharing of what was also a private family event. I remember his wife, Nancy Reagan, and the dignity with which she managed the subsequent years until his death. It struck me at the time of his farewell comments that this was a sort of prison sentence, and that not much could be done about it.

This was one of my first realizations about the powerful impact of Alzheimer's and the toll it takes on the family. To watch someone you love slip away, day by day, to witness them not be able to recall events, initially from the present and then even from the past. Eventually, to lose them altogether. More recently in 2011, Larry King did a special on Alzheimer's and interviewed the President's son, Ron Reagan. He asked him, if it were possible to know whether a person would develop the disease, would he want to know ahead of time. Ron simply said no. Perhaps, this is because, currently, there is no known cure for the disease.

## Edith

As I'd shared earlier in the introduction, my initial desire to start looking into Alzheimer's started with my own family. My stepmother, Edith, was always the one who showed me, very early in life, what kindness and courtesy looked like. After my mom and dad divorced, it was Edith, the "other woman" in my dad's life who took care of me when I would spend summers in central California. She was a beautiful, refined and calming influence for my dad. Her family lineage was from northern Italy and she was actually the first person to introduce me to cultures and traditions other than the ones I'd come to know in my youth.

Whatever shortcomings my dad had, the one thing that was clear to me was his total dedication to Edith. Over almost 50 years of marriage, he demonstrated how his partner in life was always a top priority. And so, in the later years of Edith's life when this puzzling disease made it harder and harder for him to take care of her, it finally a became necessary for Edith to move into a nursing home. Thankfully, it was located not far down the street from their home. I remember visiting her there and seeing that puzzled and blank look on her face. I could see her struggle to find some recognition of who I was, almost as though she was remembering the chubby, somewhat emotional 8-year-old who she would seat at her Aunt Stella's Italian restaurant, where they all make a fuss over me. I stood there in her room at the nursing home and remembered how Edith would stuff a metal tin full of chocolate chip cookies for me to take home when I returned to L.A. Somehow, I always thought if I could hold onto that metal tin and keep it sealed up, none of the love she had for me would ever get lost.

As time went on, my dad also lost strength and had to move into an assisted living facility, but not where Edith was staying. Initially, he was not ill enough to warrant his being at the same place. By the time he was, however, he ended up in a disorienting facility a few towns over. He passed away first, calling out for Edith, who he thought had been misplaced or lost. My brother and I, living in other states, missed the administrative oversights, until one day it was too late. One of the hard-learned lessons I can pass along here is that it is painful to watch a couple who have shared so much be unable to share their last few years in close proximity.


## Carol

Unfortunately, as I'd also shared in the introduction, my personal connection to Alzheimer's does not end there. Just a few years after Edith passed away, my sister-in-law, Carol, started to display some puzzling mental symptoms. My brother took her to a series of doctors, including the Mayo Clinic in Scottsdale. Finally, one of the neurologists there determined she was suffering from a type of brain shrinkage that was affecting her mental condition and ultimately her physical state, as well. While she was not officially diagnosed with Alzheimer's, she had all the cognitive impairment of dementia. Of course, there are some other pieces to this story, which bear mentioning. Carol had lost a son when he was in his early 30's, and it is my suspicion that this traumatic loss affected her overall mental well-being. I remember visiting her one time, and it was as if we were talking in an alternate universe. Having grown up in the 60's, this was actually not too unusual for me, and there were times when even humor could be found in the situation. However, as it happens in many cases, Carol ultimately needed much greater care than could be provided at home. She passed away just a few years ago, at a relatively early age (in her early 60's). She had been in my life since I was 12 years old and married to my brother for over 40 years. In a sense, she was a big sister to me, always supportive and loyal through some of my own tough personal times, and always putting blood and family first.

Carol also taught me about some other aspects of the Alzheimer's disease and dementia process. For example, there can be an emotional component to the process. I'm certainly not a psychologist, but I'm sure it will not be a surprise to find out that sometimes we just don't *want* to remember. We may not know how that resistance to remembering specifically affects the brain, but it is interesting to note that even some patients in nursing homes who take Aricept (one of the popular "go to" drugs for Alzheimer's) don't always like it because, at least according to some of my nursing friends, it "makes them remember."

While this is the intended result of the drug—to assist in brain function, including memories—it is not always the case, especially, if the memory is not welcome. I'll touch more on this when we discuss alternatives to treatment with advanced craniosacral techniques.

Yet another insight I learned from Carol is that not all types of dementia are labeled the same way. Some are vascular related, some are more temporal parietal, and some do not track with the classic symptoms patients typically exhibit. This was the case with Carol, as she was never conclusively diagnosed with dementia. In the main, however, about 65% of all dementia is classified as Alzheimer's, which explains why it has received such a great deal of attention. However, this also got me thinking about related causes and diseases, which then led me, unintentionally, to research how other diseases may contribute to Alzheimer's symptoms. What I've discovered is this: in many cases, dementia is just the tip of the iceberg, so to speak; so much so, that we have an entire chapter dedicated to this subject.

Finally, Carol's condition led me to understand why the condition is ultimately life-threatening and not just a "mental condition." Through continued research on the brain inflammatory processes, I began to understand how, after years of conflict within the body, the respiratory and cardiac systems begin to fail. Not at all a pleasant picture, which is why I believe some alternatives need to be investigated. Simply put, rather than watching the brain shrink and dry out, we can use techniques from CST to "re-irrigate" the brain and nervous system and improve or restore brain function.

\* \* \* \* \* \* \*

It's because of Edith and Carol that I wrote this book and undertook the research. There are many stories to follow, but it is family, for many of us, that draws us together in a common quest to understand and help others. I would like to share the following stories, as well, because they also illustrate the role of caregivers and the effect Alzheimer's and dementia may have on them.

I'd like to also extend my heartfelt thanks to Maria Shriver for all her great work in creating a website and nationwide support group for caregivers of Alzheimer's. The examples below are from her website: _www.mariashriver.com_. I suggest you read them in their entirety, when you have the time.

## Sara Pines—Caregiver

Maria mentions Sara Pines, the self-described "sandwich mom" who is raising a 5-year-old and taking care of a dad who is in the later stages of Alzheimer's. Sarah started a blog about her life. What makes this great is that it is just that, a blog. She chronicles, day-by-day, the small but significant changes she sees and has to deal with over time.

If you happen to be one who has not experienced Alzheimer's, first-hand, it would be hard for you to imagine the cumulative effects of many years of coping with a loved one who is living with this disease—all the feelings involved, the deciding, the grieving, accepting, learning, growing and coming to action. For a more in-depth look, I encourage you to read some of what Sara Pines has to say. You'll observe, as she does, that life doesn't happen in large chunks. It is a series of small realizations that culminate in a collective world view and attitude. I sincerely recommend looking to people like Sara, who can see the sweet and the bittersweet. She talks candidly about the more complicated situations that many of us are juggling, and she represents a call to how traditional and non-traditional family structures can be created to both accept and create more positive change and outcomes through the family network.

## Trish Vradenberg

Trish Vradenberg shared on Maria Shriver's website how she first came to realize her mother was in trouble. Trish's mom was one of those larger-than-life figures who seemed to be able to do anything at anytime. According to Trish, her mom could master anything, manage multiple tasks simultaneously and always be ready to handle any emergency, all the while generously giving advice to her daughter, free of charge. One day, Trish had a fall at home and realized she needed to get to the hospital. She called her mother, who lived 5 minutes away, and asked her to come over to help her. An hour later her mom pulled into the driveway. Her mom said, "Are we having tea?" and Trish looked at her in disbelief. Then her mom said, "How do you like my hat?" and Trish knew something was definitely wrong. That was the start of a slide that ended five years later, when her mother passed away.

Here are some questions to ponder, given that short, yet telling tale. "How could such a vibrant person go downhill so quickly? Is there a possibility that stress might have been a factor in her life?" We have learned that stress can lead to inflammation, which in turn can cause dysfunction in the body, which then can lead to inflammation in the brain. This series of connections brings up another quite salient question: "Could anything more have been done?"

## Karen Henley and Angie Clarkson

Both Karen and Angie describe their experience with early onset Alzheimer's on Maria Shriver's website. Karen has a husband who is 36 years old and Angie's mom is 61. Their stories illustrate that this disease isn't just for the elderly, and it made me realize that my sister-in-law was in the category of early onset Alzheimer's. In fact, most cases (approximately 80%) of Alzheimer's are seen in a population older than 60 years, showing that its development prior to 60 is fairly rare. Many Alzheimer's researchers, of course, speak about genetics, but still are puzzled by the exact mechanism of the disease. Contemplating early onset Alzheimer's, other questions naturally began to arise in my mind: "Could it be possible that certain people are more susceptible to stress than others, and therefore react differently in their bodies? Could it be that Alzheimer's is not just a function of age, even though it is thought there are more cases of Alzheimer's because people are living longer?" Perhaps we should look at dementia through the prism of "life stress" and how the nervous system deals with it.

## My Friend, Mary Ann

Closer to home, I have a friend who shared this more recent observation about her mom:

"As for my mom, aging is such an interesting process. Last night, I found myself cutting up her meat at dinner at assisted living, thinking, *She did that for me at one time.* My mom is at the point where she can't read anymore. By the time she gets her eyes focused on a word, the one next to it 'floats away,' and when it comes back into focus, she has forgotten the first one. Now, she needs someone to read to her. As I watch the slow decline of her faculties, I feel so much love and compassion for this woman who I've spent most of my life "locking horns" with. Life is so full of surprising twists and turns, isn't it?"

## One Last Personal Story: CST Action Team in Indianapolis

A student attended my 2-day class in Iowa for the prevention and treatment of Alzheimer's and dementia. Her husband was in a nursing home in Indianapolis, and was there mainly because he could not physically function well enough to be cared for at home. He also had a diagnosis of Parkinson's and a history of other health challenges, as well. I proposed to her that we send in a CST Action Team of trained therapists to work on him in an intensive way over the course of three days. I recruited four therapists—consisting of a chiropractor, a rolfer, a massage therapist and an occupational therapist—all trained in CST. The results of their afternoon visits were more than interesting. While our patient was not able to be discharged, one of the nurses working there was amazed at the improvement in his movement, ability to walk (at least 50% better) and in general, improved attitude and vitality. These results offered up yet another learning experience for us to see how teams of therapists, when appropriately managed, can turn back the clock on accumulated Alzheimer's history and actually improve the patient's quality of life. Perhaps being in a nursing home no longer has to be a one-way street.

## Chapter 4

# Dr. Upledger and the Power of Touch

My personal odyssey to discover what more could be done about Alzheimer's disease and dementia really began with Dr. John Upledger. "Dr. John" as many of us called him, was the inspiration for a new type of osteopathic work called craniosacral therapy, which we'll explore in greater detail in this chapter than we have thus far. But to arrive at a sufficiently clear understanding of craniosacral therapy, we need to trace back its origins in the field of therapeutic medicine known as osteopathy.

Osteopathy really began over a hundred years ago, developed by Andrew Taylor Still, a Civil War physician and surgeon who practiced medicine in the northern part of Missouri in the 1870's and 1880's. Having come to realize there were other ways to address chronic conditions in the body without the harmful effects of drugs, Dr. Still formulated a series of guiding therapeutic principles, and began using them in his regular practice. (These principles are still used by osteopaths today.) In 1892, inspired by his own observations, he founded the American School of Osteopathy in Kirksville, Missouri (now the A.T. Still University of the Health Sciences). Among the common beliefs of the day was the thought that the body contained a "natural pharmacy" that could help internally cure any disease process.

The influence of Dr. Still's initial work carried with it an important "ripple effect." Not only did he believe the body had an inherent wisdom that could heal itself, but he taught other doctors to apply those principles in a practical, loving and caring way to their patients. It's noteworthy that, before some major changes in the American medical profession, this emphasis on natural cures and trust in inner guidance was the standard of the day.

Dr. Still had a star student by the name of William Garner Sutherland, whom he mentored in the early 1900's. Sutherland was fascinated by the movement of the bones in the head and suggested to Dr. Still that he pursue this course of study. With Dr. Still's blessing, Sutherland spent the next few years developing a body of work that we now know as Cranial Osteopathy. Sutherland was innovative enough to study on himself, which meant he used unconventional techniques such as lacing catcher's mitts together with a series of straps and buckles placed around his own head. Although somewhat amusing to imagine, out of his work, Sutherland was able to confirm that the bones of the head actually do display a subtle motion, which has important consequences for speaking, learning, balance, coordination, emotion, memory and mental cognition.

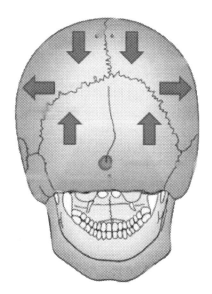

**SKULL** (Posterior View)
Skull in flexion shortens anterior and posterior, widens laterally

Even more importantly, I believe, was the work Sutherland did in developing a theory explaining how the tensions in the membranes within the brain interact with each other (a reciprocal tension membrane system) and how this contributes to a rhythmic fluctuation of cerebrospinal fluid (CSF) and venous drainage. His theories about the pumping action or fluctuation of CSF laid the groundwork for Dr. Upledger to go forward and eventually discover that the craniosacral system (a term he would eventually coin) within the body is as fundamental as the respiratory, cardiac and nervous systems.

## Dr. Upledger: Osteopath, Innovator, Healer

Dr. Upledger had an unconventional arrival into the world of medicine. He was an accomplished jazz musician, who grew up on the streets of Detroit and graduated from playing the accordion at age seven to playing piano in jazz bands as a teenager. After serving as a medical corpsman in the Coast Guard, he asked his family doctor if he thought he was smart enough to be a doctor. Fortuitously, his physician gave him the green light. Interestingly enough, it turned out the family doctor was an osteopath, and soon John Upledger was bound for Kirksville, Missouri, to start his osteopathic training.

Dr. Upledger's unique way of thinking about and looking at the body was also strongly influenced by his studies with Dr. Stacy Howell at Kirksville. Dr. Howell was a runner up for a Nobel Prize in biochemistry, and Dr. Upledger received a Rockefeller scholarship to study with him, while simultaneously getting his medical degree. In this unique collaboration, Dr. Upledger was trained to truly think "outside the box" and develop formulations and theories about the body's behavior that allowed him to see the origin of a problem and not just the symptoms.

In his continuous learning process, Dr. Upledger also began to learn about cranial osteopathy, which was, quite frankly, looked at with a fair amount of skepticism by the mainstream osteopathic community. In the mid-1970's, he was part of a research team at Michigan State University that consisted of about 20 osteopaths, scientists and other experts to examine the claims of Sutherland, and to establish if, indeed, Sutherland's approach had any basis in scientific fact. Sutherland had felt he was able to sense and intuit the movement of the cranial bones, and developed theories about the movement of cerebral spinal fluid within the brain and spinal column. It was during this research period that Dr. Upledger began to define what we now know as the craniosacral system.

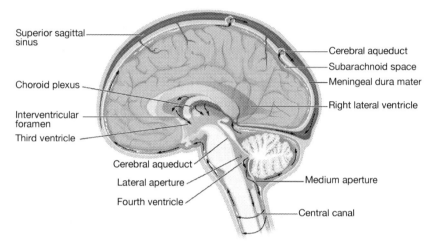

Superior sagittal sinus

Choroid plexus

Interventricular foramen

Third ventricle

Cerebral aqueduct

Lateral aperture

Fourth ventricle

Cerebral aqueduct

Subarachnoid space

Meningeal dura mater

Right lateral ventricle

Medium aperture

Central canal

While combining his anatomical knowledge and his hands-on approach to patients, Dr. Upledger began to realize that the craniosacral system was fundamental to the body. He discovered that it was an excellent way to read dysfunctions of the cardiac, respiratory and musculoskeletal system, not to mention the aberrations of the nervous system, as well. A powerful example of this was seen when he and his graduate students were visiting a school for autism. After working with these children for a few weeks, he was amazed when he found that the otherwise active and more difficult children were silently waiting at the door for his weekly visits. He then started to perceive the potential applications of his treatments to children with autism and cerebral palsy. Thirty years later, CST has become a well-established modality for the treatment of challenged infants and children.

Part of the thread that led me to suggest research on CST and Alzheimer's and dementia came from Dr. Upledger's initial research. At Michigan State in Lansing, Michigan, he developed what he called the

PressureStat model, which was a way of explaining how cerebrospinal fluid circulates throughout the central nervous system. At any one time, he found, there is about 125–150 mL, or four fluid ounces, of CSF within the body. Before getting acquainted with CST, I thought there were gallons of this fluid gushing around the body; but this is not the case. However, what is important is that this fluid is continuously circulating and is flushed throughout vital nervous system structures on a continuous basis. In the course of a day, the body produces in the range of 400–800 mL of CSF. Various research papers cite different volumes of this turnover, and conclusive testing is not currently available. So, in the interest of simplicity, I will use the average of 500–600 mL per day. This means that the body is using this fluid, absorbing it and recharging vital structures 4–5 times a day. This is called "replacement volume, as a measure of turnover of CSF."

In an article he wrote several years ago, Dr. Upledger mentioned this exchange of CSF appears to slow with age. Thus, while the complete turnover of CSF is about 4–5 times a day in healthy, middle-aged adults, this rate may be cut in half in elderly people. This focus on CSF turnover was so interesting that other researchers put shunts in the brains of some patients to study CSF turnover, to see if drainage of stagnant CSF enhances production and reduces certain substances in the CSF that may contribute to brain deterioration and Alzheimer's disease. The study mentioned above showed that the experimental group using the shunting procedure actually demonstrated a better ability to maintain cognitive function, while the control group showed a decline in cognitive function over the same time period (one year).

Additionally, other research suggests that in people with advanced Alzheimer's, where amyloid plaque is present in the brain, this plaque itself may absorb CSF and further slow its production. This finding was part of the thread that got me thinking about the impact of CSF on "at risk" seniors. I wondered how seniors could be affected by a diminished replacement volume of CSF and was curious to know if keeping the current function of the craniosacral system would improve their health.

During Dr. Upledger's research into the craniosacral system, he developed many therapeutic innovations, including the 10 Step Protocol, SomatoEmotional Release, and observations about brain structure and the immune system, especially how they relate to the craniosacral system.

However, what transcends all these therapeutic avenues is the StillPoint technique. Originally brought to light by Dr. Sutherland, the StillPoint technique allows the craniosacral system to come to a gradual and deep rest, giving the core of the nervous system an invaluable "time out" to reset and recalibrate. In terms of cerebralspinal fluid flow in the brain, resetting the nervous system with a StillPoint can have the benefit of:

- Increasing the flow of CSF, which assists in the flushing of stagnant substances within the brain; and,
- Relaxing and expanding the microscopic channels of the membrane system within the cranium—the dura mater, arachnoid mater and pia mater—which directly and indirectly increases the ability of this core system to reabsorb and more easily drain toxins and the by-products of inflammation out of the blood brain barrier. (See chart below for more health-related StillPoint benefits.)

Think of a StillPoint as hitting the reset button on a computer. When this reset occurs, it's as if the body gets a mini-craniosacral therapy treatment in just a few minutes. For this reason, I decided to use the StillPoint as a central feature in the prevention and treatment for Alzheimer's and dementia patients. This technique is easily learned and can be mastered over a one- or two-day period by laypersons, family members and healthcare practitioners alike.

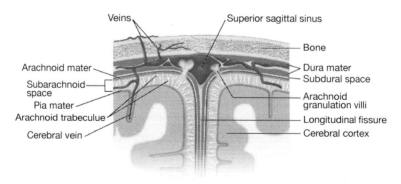

A StillPoint can be induced to help facilitate the release of restrictions in the membranes around the brain and spinal cord. One theory is that the interruption of cerebrospinal fluid flow causes a momentary buildup of fluid in the system. When the tissues are released and the cerebrospinal fluid begins to flow again, it gently flushes the system, causing the membranes to stretch a bit and release tissue restrictions or adhesions. The results include increased blood flow to the brain and can have a therapeutic effect on the central nervous system and the entire body. Some other highly beneficial effects include headache and muscle pain relief, a reduced state of stress and ready response, a deep state of relaxation, and a general sense of well-being.

### Benefits of a Stillpoint:

- Increased blood flow to the brain
- Increased flow of Cerebral Spinal Fluid
- Increased flexibility of the Central Nervous System
- Reduction of Stress
- Reduction of Blood Pressure
- Decrease in cerebral/pulmonary congestion
- Aids in removal of metabolic waste
- Reduces Headaches and Migraines
- Aids in removal of metallic toxins across the blood brain barrier

Sutherland believed that a StillPoint also increases the flow of CSF and can help to counter the effects of the aging process by keeping the brain healthy. Second, healthy CSF flow will increase the natural cleansing action, eliminating toxicity in the brain. And finally, it allows for rest and repairs to take place in the central nervous system.

Craniosacral therapy does more than just treat the membrane system, brain and nervous system. Structurally, CST allows the therapist to follow the subtle, yet profound flow of cerebral spinal fluid. The therapist can feel the effects of the rhythm throughout the body, like ripples in a pond. Found in the meningeal system of the body, lining the inside of the head and the outside of the spinal cord, this flow of CSF transfers vital neurotransmitters and other substances to the brain and spinal cord. The flow of these neurotransmitters is vital to brain health, longevity, complete mental functioning and "creativity," all of which make such a difference to the quality of one's life. While this flow is palpable, it is also very subtle, and it takes a certain amount of stillness and quietness to follow it. Dr. Upledger discovered, through his own hands, the need for the therapist to follow their own craniosacral rhythm and those of others with a very, very light touch, on the level of 5 grams, which seems more like a "baby touch" than anything else. However, there is a lot of kindness and respect that goes with this territory. This kindness and respect has translated into the teaching of over 100,000 therapists since 1985, a great many of whom have solved difficult problems for their patients, including cessation of lower back pain, PTSD, birth trauma, digestive disorders, TMJD, brain trauma and migraine headaches, to just to name a few. Often, it is the CST therapist who is successful in helping the person who has gotten to a place of giving up, so to speak, having tried "everything else."

One of the things Dr. Upledger believed in quite strongly was the self-empowerment of his patients. He discovered through his therapy that everyone has an inner wisdom, or what he called an Inner Physician, that provides guidance and well-being if one could just tune in and listen to it. While on the board of directors of an alternative medicine panel, he made a trip to Washington, DC to attend a meeting. During his stay in Washington, one of the doctors invited him to take a tour of one of the inner city schools. He ended up speaking in a high school class about his work. What he didn't realize was that this class was composed entirely of youth who had witnessed at least one murder. Talk about a tough audience! He silently asked his inner wisdom for guidance, and ended up teaching one youth, and then another, how to use their energy in a positive way to heal old aches and pains. By the end of the class the entire atmosphere had changed from anger and resentment to at least some level of love and acceptance.

Dr. Upledger came away from that experience wondering to himself, *If this could work for these teenagers, what could be the result if younger kids could learn to use their positive energy early on and help each other, and as a result, lower the level of violence in schools?* The result was the birth of the Compassionate Touch Program, which has been taught in many schools across the U.S. over the past several years.

As a compliment to this program, the Upledger Institute has promoted a class called ShareCare, which also trains adults with no healthcare background how to support each other with simple craniosacral therapy techniques. For those wanting to support their challenged children between treatments, and for those wanting to give greater comfort to their parents, these classes have been a tremendous contribution.

I'd like to mention that it is upon this foundation that the BodyEnergy Institute for Longevity and Quality of Life has created a two-day class entitled "CranioSacral Therapy for Longevity: Applications for the Treatment of Alzheimer's and Dementia." This class is specifically designed to train and support adult children of Alzheimer's or at risk parents, and also caregivers in this situation. Again, the concept is very simple: empower the patient, empower the family, empower those who come in daily contact with those who are the most fragile and at the greatest risk.

This concludes our brief overview of Dr. John Upledger and the development of modern craniosacral therapy. There is more to come about his contributions to the field of health in the following chapters. Dr. Upledger passed away in the latter part of 2012. He was a great mentor to many of us, and in a way, his life purpose can be summarized in a simple phrase, which was: "to help people." I feel he has done so much more than that. He has laid the groundwork for an entire generation to potentially shift the outcome of how we look at our health and the body's response, especially as it relates to the disease process known as Alzheimer's. Thank you, Dr. John.

Chapter **5**

# Inflammation and the Brain

In researching the causes and development leading to Alzheimer's and dementia, I've had the unique advantage of following Dr. Upledger's advanced research on the immune system response and the inflammatory processes in the brain. In addition to Dr. Upledger's fundamental contribution to the field of osteopathy in developing a contemporary version of the craniosacral system as discussed in the last chapter, he continued to add to the academic and therapeutic field by developing the concept of SomatoEmotional Release and offering his observations about how to use imagery and dialogue with different parts of the brain and specific cellular structures within the immune system. I'll be discussing a few of these concepts in this chapter, as we look at the human brain's inflammatory mechanism, which offers a possible explanation for how Alzheimer's and dementia take root in the brain.

It's worth noting, here, that contemporary scientific research references these inflammatory mechanisms, as well. A number of articles in the *Journal of the Neurological Sciences* can be found mentioning the pro-inflammatory response and neurotoxicity. Additionally, researchers in *Psychiatry Online* discuss inflammatory mechanisms that have been associated with Alzheimer's disease.

Let's start with the basics and look at how the body develops an inflammatory response, in the first place. The immune system is designed to protect us from intrusion, especially from 'outside' factors that may compromise the normal functioning of the body. Immune system cells are constantly scanning the body for signs of anything suspicious or unlike the normal cells found in the body. In a very real sense the immune system is always distinguishing 'self' from 'non-self.' When the immune system identifies anything that is perceived as a threat, oftentimes, depending on the level of the threat, other immune system cells 'rush in' to attack, digest, poison or otherwise eliminate the intruder. The result is what we call the inflammatory response.

If you've ever sprained your ankle or had an insect bite or a bee sting, you know how the body can swell up and get puffy around the sprain or swell up and develop a bright red area around the bite. This 'swelling up' is an indication of the inflammatory response at work. We can look at this as an irritation or aggravation to the body, which in a sense it is; but what is actually going on is the body is both eliminating a threat and, in the process, carting off waste products and toxicity that are a by-product of this response. We oftentimes observe this as swelling and puffiness. Ultimately, we can think of an inflammatory response as the immune system's way of defending and purifying itself.

In and of itself, an inflammatory response is not "a bad thing." When it becomes prolonged, sustained or chronic, however, problems can arise.

It's important to realize the body will always want to respond appropriately, and often, nature has equipped us with a way to isolate or 'splint' an injury, to give the body at least a temporary respite to rest and repair. As the saying goes, "Mother Nature knows best," and mechanisms in our bodies will make us take the time to slow down even if we have other ideas about what we want to do. Many would say that this is the way we have adapted and survived as a species. However, the problem that starts to develop is that, after a certain 'time out' period, usually within 48–96 hours, the body starts to adapt in an unnatural and unhealthy way to this emergency inflammation reaction. Let's look, now, into how this adaptive mechanism can lead to further problems piling up in the body and brain.

It may seem obvious, but there is an intimate connection between this inflammatory response and the body's immune system. In the example of the bee sting mentioned above, certain immune system cells known as mast cells begin to overproduce, involving a histamine reaction that is like an army going on a massive attack. If the immune system is not properly regulated, overreaction of this type can cause problems not intended by the body. In the case of an allergic reaction to bee stings, it can result in death. This example is on the extreme end of the immune response spectrum, but it *does* illustrate why the regulation, management and gentle (or not so gentle) urging of the immune system has occupied the attention of the pharmaceutical industry for the past several decades.

When examining some of the "key players" in the immune system that react to and regulate this inflammatory response, you can think of them like a football team going out onto the field, with the players and coaches taking action and providing guidance, respectively, as the game unfolds. Research professor Dr. Lauren Sompayrac, author of *How the Immune System Works,* uses this analogy of players, coaches and quarterbacks to explain how the immune system responds to a threat. In his analogy, the innate immune system (basic to all animals) is constantly scanning for evidence of any foreign intrusion in the body. He likens the innate immune system to the 'coach' of the immune system. If the coach detects anything that looks like a threat, he/she delivers to the quarterback (in this case, helper T-cells, part of the adaptive immune system) a game plan that directs the adaptive immune system into appropriate action. The adaptive immune system is a more specialized form of the immune system, and chooses which weapons are needed to eliminate the threat, and where and how to send them (the players).

When dealing with Alzheimer's, however, at least as far as past and current medical models have been concerned, you should realize the "team" has always ended up losing tragically (i.e., the patient dies). The point to be made is that our immune system involves a coordinated effort, good communication and a response that can be predictable or unexpected. However, if you'll follow this through with me, you'll discover—as did I—some practical, effectual options that can deliver an alternate, more desirable result.

In terms of inflammation in the brain and inflammation in the body, in general, I'd like to provide you with a quick overview of the key elements that are typically involved in this response. Mind you, this is not meant to be a detailed overview, but it will hopefully be sufficient for you to appreciate the BodyEnergy theory of how the brain is affected by inflammation. To begin, I'll describe how the immune system organizes itself into the various components.

## Layers of Protection

### The Skin and Digestive System

If any of you are science fiction fans, you are familiar with the concept of a "shield" as a defensive barrier to an attack. Our skin is our outer layer shield, covering our body and forming the primary defensive barrier between us and the outside world, protecting us, in many ways, from harm. The other "layer of protection," at this level of defense, is our digestive system, as reflected in the mucous membranes that line our gut, which actually cover hundreds of times more square feet than our outer skin lining. Think of the mucous membranes as the inner folds of the skin, but inside the body. They interface with other substances brought in from outside the body, in this case, food. Their job is to help in the processes of both absorption and digestion, which provides vital and necessary energy to the body. Additionally, and this is the protective function, the mucous membranes help sort out what is usable and what is toxic to the body. (As an aside, the immune system literally underlies this lining of the digestive system, which may go a long way in explaining how what we eat and how we digest it may influence the immune system's response.)

### The Innate Immune System

On both the skin and the inner lining of the digestive system, not to mention other parts of our bodies, lies our second layer of defense, the innate immune system. One of two major divisions of the immune system (the other being the *adaptive* immune system, which we'll discuss shortly), it is designed to protect us from bacteria, parasites, and a variety of foreign bodies. Innate means that something is "inborn," so this part of the immune system is a very instinctual defense system that reacts in a very predictable and intelligent way, using a variety of cells to protect us. Among the components of the innate immune system that are thought to play a role in the inflammatory response are:

1.  *Stem Cells*

Stem cells are where the immune system begins. These amazing entities can reproduce both themselves and all of the other blood cells in the body—hence the name "stem." Dr. Upledger felt that stem cells could be induced to repair many of the cells in the body that had been damaged at some point. We'll talk more about the significance of stem cells in a later chapter.

2.  *Phagocytes*

These are cells that protect by virtue of their ability to digest foreign agents in the body. There are many types of phagocytes, two of these being the monocyte and macrophage discussed below. Others include neutrophils, basophils, eosinophils and natural killer cells.

3.  *Monocytes*

Monocytes are found in the blood and work to keep the blood clean. However, they can move quickly to the site of an infection. Once they enter the tissue, they can then become and adapt to being a type of cell required to trigger the immune response. Often this is a macrophage. This adaptability of monocytes is important to our discussion of brain inflammation, since monocytes are said to be one of the immune system factors that can cross the blood brain barrier and become involved in the process of the inflammatory response.

4.  *Macrophages*

The macrophage, one of the primary lines of defense of the innate immune system, literally means "big eater," and they will digest anything seen as an intruder.

5.  *Cytokines*

Cytokines (from the Greek "cyto" for cell and "kinos" for movement) are proteins that are created by a broad range of cells—especially immune system cells—in response to a threat. They literally "communicate" between macrophages and other cells to bring the reinforcements to a site where more help is needed. Two classes of cytokines, inflammatory and anti-inflammatory, help support the response of the immune system to an emergency reaction. These messengers help to increase production of proteins in the cells, which can then be used to combat or promote inflammation. As always, it's a matter of the appropriate measure of response. When there is a continuous triggering and demand for cytokines as pro-inflammatories, the body itself starts to create its own hot spots or toxicity.

Please take a look at the chart below for an overview of how important cytokines are to the immune system. Dr. Upledger felt that cytokines, especially the pro-inflammatory variety, play a key role in how both the body and the brain react to a threat. They can, however, create an *ongoing* response that can be detrimental. If left unchecked, they can spur an ever-increasing spiral of inflammatory response. We'll discuss more about the role of these pro-inflammatory cytokines when we outline the BodyEnergy theory of the brain's inflammatory response.

## Questions and Answers About Cytokines

**What are cytokines?**
*They are molecular messengers between cells.*

**What are they made of?**
*Cytokines are proteins produced by cells.*

**What do they do?**
*Cytokines interact with cells of the immune system in order to regulate the body's response to disease and infection. Cytokines also mediate normal cellular processes in the body.*

### Types of Cytokines:
*Some cytokines stimulate production of blood cells, which is a good thing and can function as a back up to the immune system. There are also some that regulate other cell population, monitoring their maturation, growth and responsiveness. And then there are some that are immunoregulatory, pro-inflammatory and anti-inflammatory.*

*It is the pro-inflammatory cytokines that cause such potential damages to the brain. In moderate to severe Alzheimer's, examples of these pro-inflammatories are:*

- *Colony stimulating factors*
- *IL-1*
- *TNF-tumor necrosis factor*

6. *Natural Killer (NK) T-Cells*

NK T-cells deserve a brief mention here. These cells have the special ability of injecting a poison to kill an "invader." Working in tandem with macrophages, these cells provide a significant contribution to the formidable defense of the innate immune system. Incidentally, NK T-cells are part of both the innate and adaptive immune systems.

## The Adaptive Immune System

As the name implies, the adaptive immune system has the ability to adapt itself to specific threats, especially in the case of viruses that sneak into a cell and thereby avoid detection by the innate immune system. In addition, the innate immune system can put out an alert, sort of like an "all points bulletin," to inform the adaptive immune system of potential threats it could not effectively deal with on its own. In that sense, the adaptive immune system is our third line of defense. A few of its key components are described below:

1. *Thymus*

This small, but important organ of the immune system is located in front of the heart and behind the sternum. It is considered by some to play a significant role in the "education" of the adaptive immune system. Dr. Upledger likened the thymus to a master librarian that gathers the history of what the body has encountered (from a bacterial or viral point of view) and informs the appropriate cells about which components are self (native) and which are non-self (foreign). The job, then, of these cells is to constantly scan the body for any signs of intruders that may not be part of the makeup of the body. Current neurological research now tells us that the thymus helps create a more customized response to a threat, using DNA recombination to look for only one threat at a time. In a sense, this would represent a more efficient response to a variety of threats, and would use significantly less "memory," on a cellular level.

2. *T-Cells*

Manufactured in the thymus, there are a few varieties of T-cells: helper, killer and adaptive. Dr. Lauren Sompayrac, the distinguished immune system researcher, describes the helper T-cells as "the quarterback" of the immune system, helping to create cytokine factories that can respond to an emergency. Another example of T-cells in action occurs when specific viruses or threats bypass the innate immune system. Killer T-cells are then able to penetrate into the body of a cell to eliminate the threat. The adaptive T-cells, whose function is not clearly understood, seem to help regulate the response of all these T-cells.

3.   *B-Cells*

Related to the bone marrow, B-cells play a vital role in helping to create special proteins called *antibodies,* which then produce corresponding antigens to protect us from specific viral threats. What is amazing about these B-cells is that they are modular in design and can, on demand, respond to over 100 million possible combinations of viral threats, as needed. Actually, in 1987, a Nobel Prize was awarded to Susumu Tonegawa who identified how the genetics of the immune system can mix and match a genetic response to a wide variety of threats.

Now that we've discussed some of the key components of the immune system, I'd like to share with you my theory of how brain inflammation advances in Alzheimer's patients. This perspective is based on Dr. Upledger's observation of the reversal of the pathogenic process, my own observations of immune system response in the brain, and other commentators in the field of geriatric neurology.

I'll like to start by saying that immune system activity in the central nervous system, and especially in the brain, is *not* the typical state of affairs. It takes something unusual and chronic to trigger a reaction that results in ongoing and persistent inflammation in the brain. One of the many possible contributors to this situation is insulin resistance, which left untreated can result in diabetes. I mention this because studies have shown that 40–43% of all Alzheimer's patients also have diabetes. How is such a high percentage possible?

Insulin helps glucose (sugar) get into the cells. When this process becomes ineffective, it results in glucose remaining outside the cells, which then can lead to a state of chronic inflammation. (Some have likened diabetes to having cells that are drowning in a sea of plenty.) Notice I use the word "chronic."

What causes this process to become ineffective, and therefore creates insulin resistance, is persistent, ongoing exposure to high concentrations of sugar. Persistent is the key word here. Sugar is natural and useful for the body, at least in small concentrations. However, what has occurred over the years is that more and more sugar has been added to so many of our foods—obviously because sugar (as well as salt and fats) makes food taste better, a fact not lost on the food industry. The problem is, to quote functional medicine expert, Dr. Karyn Shanks: "High concentrations of sugar can be toxic." That is, the digestive system can process and use relatively low concentrations of sugar safely; but when exposed to high concentrations over a prolonged period to time, the body can start to 'reject' it, becoming unable to absorb the excess concentration. Those higher concentrations, over time, can lead to the body's developing an adaptive inflammatory response—and unfortunately the brain reflects these higher concentrations of sugar and insulin resistance. The onset of this inflammatory process can then set in motion the beginning of dementia.

In other words, once chronic inflammation is in place, the ground is set for it to make its way to the brain, which can then lead to dementia and Alzheimer's.

One question I see as important to consider here is: "What potential causes are there for the other 60% of Alzheimer's patients who are not diabetic?" We can divide this single large group up into many smaller groups, according to the numerous other possible causes: those who are pre-diabetic (not officially diabetic, but still carrying many of the risk factors that can generate chronic inflammation), genetic factors, age, gender (approximately 2 to 3 times more women are affected), specific genetic markers or genotypes, stress, prior trauma or injury to the body, a prior history of inflammatory diseases, and any number of toxic agents absorbed by the body over decades.

Regardless of the cause, the common theme to the BodyEnergy theory of the formation of dementia and Alzheimer's is chronic inflammation that has overflowed into the brain. I've divided this observation about inflammation in the brain into 3 stages, which loosely correspond to the classic 3 stages of Alzheimer's (early, middle and late stages).

## Stages of Inflammation:
## The Brain Inflammatory Response

### Stage 1

Recall the monocytes, which are part of the immune system defense. Monocytes are flexible and small enough to cross the blood brain barrier. If they detect even early signs of toxicity or a raised level of inflammation in the brain, they can quickly transform into macrophages, which join into the battle to protect any part of the body, including the brain. Part of the response that macrophages may elicit is to produce pro-inflammatory cytokines, which elicit an even more intensified response from the immune system. This can result in even greater inflammation. At this stage, obvious signs of dementia may not be visible. However, if left unchecked, sustained levels of inflammation can be the ground for further problems to develop.

### Stage 2

The presence of these macrophages and pro-inflammatory cytokines in the brain can lead to what is called the acute phase response. Essentially, this means the brain reacts to the continued inflammation by changing liver function, among other things, and producing even more pro-inflammatory cytokines when the response is excessive or prolonged. Now, here is a key point in this theory: in a manner that is not clearly understood (see the chapter on current research on Alzheimer's), the amalyoid precursor protein (APP) becomes compromised with the result that shorter proteins are produced, called tau, beta and gamma peptides. My theory is that this baseline of an inflammatory environment provides sufficient disorganization to result in the breakdown of APP. These amyloid peptides (especially the beta variety) form neurofibrillary tangles and amyloid plaques that are the hallmark indicator of Alzheimer's disease. In this second phase of early plaque formation, we could expect to see some of the early or moderate signs of Alzheimer's.

### Stage 3

As this formation of amyloid plaques and tangles continues, the brain starts to attack itself in an attempt to distinguish and protect itself from any and all foreign invaders. One way to describe this condition is

# BodyEnergy Model of
# Brain Inflammatory Response

STAGE ONE

Toxicity in the blood crosses the blood-brain barrier, creates an inflammatory response

Acute phase response: Pro-inflammatory cytokines react to inflammation and increase their response

STAGE TWO

This inflammatory condition and baseline toxicity interferes with normal synthesis of APP

Beta amyloidal plaques and neuro-fibular tangles start to form

STAGE THREE

Plaques and tangles are seen as foreign material and invaders by the immune system

Inflammatory chemicals increase and the immune system begins to "digest" the brain

Continued destruction of healthy and unhealthy brain tissue continues chronic immune activation. Cells in the brain called microglia recognize the plaque as an invader. They, in turn, produce inflammatory chemicals (cytokines) in an attempt to clear out the amyloid. However, in this third stage, the microglia are unable to clear out the plaque, and what is left is a backlog of amyloid and inflammatory chemicals in the brain. Dr. Upledger believed that at this point immune system factors—such as macrophages and phagocytes—begin to digest both healthy and unhealthy brain tissue. In essence, he characterized this situation as an autoimmune response in the brain, in the sense that the brain cannot recognize itself from the by-products of inflammation. Autopsies of Alzheimer's patients reflect this extensive damage, in that a great majority of brain tissue appears to be destroyed and non-functional.

## Chapter 6

# A Simple Idea Leads to a Breakthrough Study

As I mentioned in the Introduction and Chapter 3, my step-mother and sister-in-law had a significant effect on exposing me to Alzheimer's and dementia on a personal level. Those heart-rending experiences were the first steps leading to my explorations of what is possible in the treatment and care of Alzheimer's and dementia. In the last chapter, I shared some background description and possible insights into the disease, in relation to the inflammatory response. And I want you to know that, even with the talk of unchecked brain inflammation or an autoimmune response in the brain, it is not all bad news. There is a light at the end of the tunnel.

A study was designed by Dr. Linda Gerdner of Stanford University and Dr. Laura Hart of the University of Iowa to identify the effect of inducing a StillPoint (recall Dr. William Sutherland's therapeutic technique in Chapter 4) on the agitation behaviors of people with dementia. When asked by Drs. Gerdner and Hart for my collaboration, I agreed and provided the delivery of the StillPoint intervention. The study was designed to assess how the StillPoint technique, delivered every day for 6 weeks, might effect agitation in persons with dementia. A relatively well-known agitation inventory was used to evaluate agitation behaviors three weeks before the intervention, during the intervention, and three weeks post-intervention of a daily StillPoint induction.

A number of years ago, Dr. Upledger wrote an article about cerebrospinal fluid and the exchange rate of this fluid in younger and older adults. He mentioned that as a consequence of the natural aging process, older or elderly adults may have a diminished production of CSF—about half that of a normal healthy, middle-aged adult. For some reason, this caught my eye as I was becoming interested in the relationship between craniosacral therapy and Alzheimer's and dementia. An associate of mine, Dr. Laura Hart, mentioned above, discovered in her research that in people with senile dementia, the fluid flow (daily turnover of CSF) was even less than Dr. Upledger had estimated: a CSF production rate of 50–75% less than normal adults. At the time, I thought this was a significant finding.

**THE MENINGES**

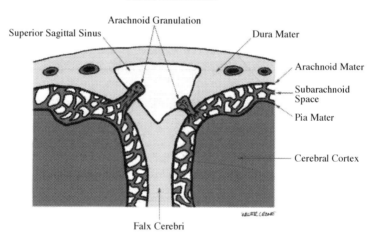

I then started to investigate the beneficial effects of cerebrospinal fluid, especially focusing on the positive effects of full and normal CSF circulation in the body. I also began looking at the effects of having *less* than normal CSF circulation.

## The Function of Cerebrospinal Fluid

For starters, cerebrospinal fluid has a chelating action. It removes waste products across the blood-brain barrier—including metallic toxins such as mercury and aluminum—through the flushing action of the

CSF. In Chapter 4, I discussed how the body creates cerebrospinal fluid and mentioned that it is then absorbed by the body. All of this creates a pumping action that Dr. Upledger called the "craniosacral rhythm." He suggested the mechanism of this, using a concept he called the "pressurestat model." More recent research suggests there is a secondary mechanism in this production and reabsorption of CSF. This secondary mechanism is reflected by research on glymphatics (a newly discovered system, by which the brain removes waste), which suggests that only 40% of the CSF flow is global and that the rest takes place locally at the blood-brain barrier. I'll discuss this in greater detail in Chapter 11, where I propose a method and approach to treat and ideally reverse the effects of Alzheimer's. This "news" about glymphatics is a potentially significant observation, and may yet explain how local repair and rejuvenation is possible, due to access of CSF at sites within the brain. This would mean there may be a global coordination of the flow of CSF, but additional local support is necessary to help promote further detoxification of the brain.

## The Implications of Reduced Cerebrospinal Fluid

• Reduced CSF flow impacts the circulation of immune system factors such as monocytes which regularly patrol the brain looking for invaders, inflammatory or otherwise

• Various immune system factors naturally try to protect the brain from foreign intrusion. One of these are amyloid precursor proteins (APP). When APP's become dysfunctional they become amyloid beta peptide which interrupt the delivery of neurotransmitter substances to the synapses of the brain

• Once dysfunction is established, the immune system reads these amyloid beta peptides (a primary component of amyloid plaques) as intruders or invaders leading to further deterioration of brain tissue

• As a response, the immune system mobilizes and creates more pro-inflammatory cytokines which creates a cycle of inflammation

The flow of CSF can be monitored by "listening" to the craniosacral rhythm (CSR) with your hands. When the therapist is evaluating the CSR, he or she is monitoring:

1.  Rate (the number of cycles per minute), amplitude (how strong the rhythm is), quality (how healthy it feels) and symmetry (whether or not it's the same in both sides of the body)

2.  Inherent energy (also known as chi, life force or prana)

3.  Circulation and non-circulation of CSF within the craniosacral system

In light of what I discovered doing research about the immune system and the inflammatory processes, the link between full, normal flow of CSF and reduced flow seemed significant. I reasoned this distinction might have a major effect on the quality of life and the diseases of aging. I then thought, *Is there any way to increase this reduced flow in people with Alzheimer's and dementia, perhaps to the level of normal adults, and is there some way we could study it?*

That's when a simple idea came to me: the key technique of craniosacral therapy (StillPoint) might help improve CSF flow. I thought, *If a StillPoint could boost the production of CSF, could that potentially solve a variety of problems for Alzheimer's and dementia?* Indirectly, I realized we can infer the beneficial effects of a StillPoint by observing the improvements cited in the initial pilot study on the craniosacral Still-Point and its effect on dementia (Gerdner, L., et al. 2008).

Certainly, I knew that further study was (and is) warranted. I was inspired to submit for publication the BodyEnergy Institute's collection of case history data, as we had treated (and continue to treat) a portion of this challenged population. After all, Dr. Sutherland, one of the aforementioned pioneers of cranial osteopathy, called it "the shotgun technique"—mainly because he observed that it addressed a wide variety of symptoms. Some of us who teach this technique refer to it as a "mini-craniosacral treatment," because in 5 minutes it treats such a full range of problems.

Put another way, one of the main advantages of full and vibrant CSF flow is that it creates a washing action in the brain, thus avoiding the build-up of materials, including immune system waste products and toxins, which over time can lead to the formation of plaques and tangles. As was mentioned earlier, it is well-known in the medical field that plaques and tangles are some of the leading markers of Alzheimer's and dementia.

## Effects of the StillPoint

My twenty years of experience as a CST therapist and the decades of experience of thousands of CST therapists all over the world have demonstrated that a StillPoint can be induced to help facilitate the release of restrictions in the membranes around the brain and spinal cord. The interruption of cerebrospinal fluid flow causes a momentary buildup of fluid in the system. When the tissues are released and the cerebrospinal fluid begins to flow again, it gently flushes the system, causing the membranes to stretch a bit and release tissue restrictions or adhesions.

The effects or benefits of a StillPoint can include increased blood flow to the brain and a therapeutic effect on the central nervous system and the entire body. Some other beneficial effects include headache and muscle pain relief, a reduced state of stress, a deep state of relaxation, and a general sense of well-being, which affects the aging process by keeping the brain healthy. As was previously mentioned, healthy CSF flow will increase the body's natural cleansing action (including in the brain), contributing to the elimination of toxicity. Inducing a StillPoint also increases the flow of CSF and can help to counter the influence of detrimental immune system overreactions in the brain. And finally, therapeutic StillPoint treatment naturally allows for rest and repairs to take place in the central nervous system. All of these benefits, I believed (and *do* believe), taken together as a whole, will translate into a positive effect for patients living with Alzheimer's and dementia.

## A Research Study is Born

Now that I had a concept of what CST could do to help Alzheimer's and dementia, I needed to formulate a plan and see if any research could be done. I realized that I would need to work within existing care facilities and utilizing current caregivers. So, in conjunction with Dr. Laura Hart, a Professor Emeritus of Nursing at the University of Iowa, we began to ask, "What are some aspects of Alzheimer's patients' conditions that are relatively easy to measure in a nursing home environment?" In addition, we pondered, "What behaviors of Alzheimer's patients would be beneficial for them to improve?" From these questions, we developed and wrote the initial proposal for a research study on CST and Alzheimer's.

It turns out that "agitation" is one of the leading answers to both of the questions above. Alzheimer's and dementia patients can get agitated, which for the nursing staff *and* patients require a lot of time and supervision. So with a plausible variable to measure, I now had a simple place to start. Basically, the study was designed to assess how the StillPoint technique, practiced at the same time every day for 12 weeks, might impact agitation. We used a relatively well-known survey to evaluative agitation and the behavior of patients before, during, and after the intervention of the StillPoint techniques.

## Research Study

A pilot study was funded by the University of Iowa, College of Nursing, Geronotological Nursing Interventions Research Center, with additional funds coming from Hartford Centers of Geriatric Nursing Excellence, a private foundation.[2] The patients enrolled in the study were those with moderate to severe symptoms of dementia. Certified Nursing Assistants CNAs) trained in using the observation inventory rated the participants on a daily basis, regarding physical aggressive and physically nonaggressive agitation, as well as verbal agitation.

A StillPoint was induced for each of the patients each morning of the study by a certified craniosacral therapist (CST). The usual time

---

[2] The study noted above was published in the *American Journal of Gerontological Nursing*, 34(3), 2008, p 36–45 entitled, "CranioSacral StillPoint Technique-Exploring Its Effects in Individuals with Dementia" (Gerdner et al).

needed was 5 minutes (the range of time was 30 seconds to 10 minutes). There were significant reductions in all categories, many continuing into the post-intervention stages. Both certified nursing staff and family members noted these positive changes, as well. As a result of the CST treatment, the study showed, cognitive abilities were improved for some of the patients, and communication for others.

Here are some of the reasons why this study is important. Again, these are my observations and can be considered as my individual interpretation and commentary on the results:

1. The study shows the results are clinically and statistically significant. "Clinical significance" means there are practical advantages or gains for those both working and living in a nursing home environment. "Statistically," this means the results are more than a coincidence.

2. Our research also shows that the effects of the intervention—in this case, the StillPoint technique—lasted even after the treatment, for some weeks after the study.

3. There are further implications—when we increase the flow of CSF—about what I suggest the StillPoint achieves. Within the brain, we are increasing CSF flow, which helps to decrease the potential for pro-inflammatory cytokines to form, and because of this, increased flow minimizes immune system factors in an area where they are not normally required. Within the body, enhanced functioning of the craniosacral system indirectly has a positive effect on the immune system and other systems of the body. This, in turn, can have a positive effect on digestion, regulation of blood sugars and even the tendency of these patients to develop diabetes, which is suspected by some to occur in 40% of Alzheimer's patients. Again, this points out how there is an intimate interplay of both brain and body in this process of promoting wellness. Alzheimer's disease alone is such an important topic that I'll devote the next chapter into looking at it and other diseases that affect patients, even decades before the onset of Alzheimer's.

I also want to share some of the more subjective observations that were noticed during the study and reported in the above article. As a result of the StillPoint technique treatments, a 100-year-old lady changed from single word responses to speaking again in complete sentences. Another woman regained the ability to feed herself. Nursing home personnel observed that the subjects began to more easily recognize family and loved ones during their visits, which resulted in increased satisfaction for those visiting the facility. Also, nursing assistants noticed that it was easier to manage the residents. In facilities where Alzheimer's and dementia patients reside, agitation is a significant factor in the management of residents, and it can take a significant amount of time to calm and reassure residents that everything is safe and secure. The results of our study indicate CST offers a great potential for reducing agitation in patients with Alzheimer's worldwide.

Clinically, there was another observation I found both interesting and important. The effects of craniosacral therapy, over time, are cumulative, meaning that changes tend to gain momentum as time goes on. In this study, the StillPoint technique was administered at the same time every day (mid-morning) for 6 weeks consecutively. At about three weeks into the study, some of the changes mentioned were noted. The effect of a StillPoint is to free restrictions in the brain and central nervous system, as well as the rest of the body. As the flushing action of CSF increases, and the volume of CSF reaching the brain increases, there is literally less inflammation and congestion in the brain tissue. During the study, what the craniosacral practitioner subjectively observed was that the patients were able to "release restrictions" in their body and mind, layer by layer. Many craniosacral clients' faces, after sessions, looked more relaxed and energetic. It is not uncommon for a patient to look *years* younger after a treatment.

As with all scientific research, the ability to replicate findings gives more confidence in the outcome and greater power to the initial research. That's why the above study should be used as a template for further research. One of the ideas we will expand upon in later chapters is the concept of case studies that further document our initial findings. Although this is not as scientifically rigorous as the original research study, it will still be useful in supporting the initial study. I am in the process of designing an online case study template that can be used by nursing homes and other facilities to document the results of the StillPoint techniques, when applied on a daily basis. The more we can support this type of documentation, the greater the momentum will build for utilizing a cost-effective and noninvasive technique in these types of environments, both nationwide and worldwide.

This may seem like a lofty goal. But history has proven it is possible to change medical and scientific attitudes. It just takes time. As an example, we can look at the use of tobacco. Believe it or not, in the 1930's and 1940's, the use of tobacco was thought to be beneficial and a recommended treatment for high-stress patients. During this period of time, case studies were initiated to document the suspected harmful effects of tobacco use. Of course, it took decades for the research to document that tobacco was indeed harmful to one's health, and even longer for the word to get out to the general public. But eventually it did, and it was the many case studies that led the way.

In order to teach this technique in facilities, a specific format is required with the following goals:

1. Generating case studies in a facility-by-facility format. The idea is that every time a CST therapist goes into a nursing home to practice the StillPoint and other CST techniques, they start to observe and write up a case history, whether it be on one person or a group of patients. This will start to generate a body of evidence that can be referenced to the next group of nursing homes and assisted living facilities, which will especially be useful in approaching the large chain national facilities. As a subset of this, we would also invite people treating at home with family to participate.

2. Replicating the original research in an expanded and larger field, with a greater number of patients and more facilities.

3. Expanding on the original concept using more sophisticated imaging technologies and techniques. One of the popular buzz words in the current research community is "amyloid load" or the amount of potential amyloid plaques and tangles that have accumulated in the brain. If one were able to image this

amyloid load in mid- to late-stage Alzheimer's using MRI or other imaging, and compare the before and after images (after the utilization of StillPoint and other BodyEnergy techniques), there could be the potential for even more concrete verification of the effectiveness of our noninvasive solution.

In summary, I hope to expand on this case study concept and to replicate the original study in a more expanded manner, as well as use other techniques to verify the findings. However, as I have discussed in the opening chapters, the need is urgent and countless lives can be impacted by immediate, positive and constructive action. I will explore some of the options of such in the next chapter.

Chapter **7**

# The Tip of the Iceberg

When I began the study on Alzheimer's and dementia, I thought it would be enough to just trace the fairly complex ideas about brain inflammation. After all, it is a lot to absorb all the ins and outs of each thread, attempting to explain how this debilitating disease comes to pass and what might be responsible for the gradual and seemingly inevitable decline of the heath of so many seniors.

But that was not to be the case. As in many areas of research, and certainly in the case of Dr. Upledger, coincidence and happenstance often occur, which take you in a direction not initially anticipated. I began to look at all the pieces of this disease, and realized it was not as straightforward as I thought. And thus, I had to start putting all the clues together, much like you do when reading a mystery novel, to realize that Alzheimer's and dementia are really just the tip of the dysfunctional iceberg.

In 2006, I was simply observing the patients as they were being treated by our therapists. After two or three visits to the facility where we were treating (in Clinton, Iowa), it occurred to me one day, with permission from the appropriate personnel, to take a look at some of the medical records of those we were treating. I then asked the coordinator of our study, Dr. Linda Gerdner, herself at expert in the area of dementia, if any of the patients had any prior medical history. She looked at me in disbelief. "Of course!" she said.

It turned out that in most cases, patients there with moderate to severe Alzheimer's had had *decades* of medical problems, including diabetes, heart disease, osteoporosis, arthritis and a number of related issues. It may have been obvious to our chief research investigator, but it was news to me.

A few years later, in 2011, while in Southern California, I was presenting my first two-day class called "Craniosacral Therapy and Longevity: Treatment for Patients with Alzheimer's and Dementia." It was there that I heard (from one of the directors of the Southern California Alzheimer's Association) what I mentioned in an earlier chapter, that 40% of the people in Alzheimer's units have diabetes! Over the next year, as I also mentioned earlier, I began to ask other healthcare practitioners who took care of residents in nursing homes (including those where I observed them dispensing drugs of various types and descriptions) about their experiences and observations, and how they compared to this statement. I could see them mentally counting the beds of the residents, doing a roll call in their heads, and then saying, "You know, that sounds about right."

The more time went by and the more I considered these discussions, the more I truly felt some connection existed. And I was about to find some more answers. As I was writing about brain inflammation and immune system response, an associate of mine in the Northwest suggested I take a look at a book entitled, *The Blood Sugar Solution* by a young, innovative MD by the name of Mark Hyman. It turns out that Dr. Hyman had been a chief exponent of a new branch of medical research called functional medicine, which I later came to realize was very complimentary to craniosacral therapy and Dr. Upledger's approach. Dr. Hyman has since become well-known as a doctor and consultant for former President Bill Clinton, who wholeheartedly endorses Mark and his innovative medical approach.

## Diabetes

Dr. Hyman and other researchers have for some time been speaking about Alzheimer's as "type 3 diabetes." *What in the world is the connection there?* I wondered. It turns out the breadcrumbs led me back to the immune system and the inflammatory response (which I discussed in some detail in the chapter on brain inflammation).

First, let's start by describing the mechanism of diabetes…but *that* means I must take a slight detour into yet *another* concept Dr. Hyman discusses: "insulin resistance."

# Dysfunctions of the Aging Process

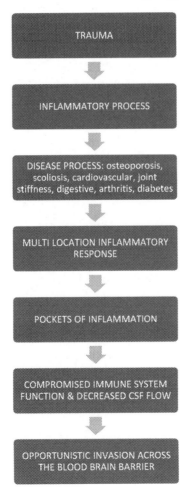

After looking at Dr. Upledger's comments on brain inflammation and Dr. Hyman's comments on diabetes and Alzheimer's as type 3 diabetes, it became clear to me that there are three aspects of Dr. Hyman's comments that are interconnected: type 3 diabetes, diabesity, and insulin resistance. Let's start with insulin resistance. Insulin resistance is a term known by most doctors, but is not commonly viewed as a precursor to diabetes, despite the fact that tests can be done to determine the level of resistance. Think of insulin resistance as the body (in particular the pancreas, which naturally produces insulin) drowning in a sea of plenty. As the body absorbs more and more sugars, the molecular mechanism in the cells begins to develop a resistance to producing or asking for more insulin from the pancreas. Part of this insulin resistance, I believe, results from an inflammatory response the body develops from digesting certain types of foods. Remember those "VIP's" (vaso-active intestinal peptides) we discussed earlier in relation to brain inflammation? They are a reflection and indication of the link between the digestive and immune system. In actuality, 70% of the immune system underlies the substrata of the digestive system. The net result is that Alzheimer's may actually, in some cases, begin *because the body is unable to metabolize sugars that are there to fuel it.* The result is toxicity around the cells, which then leads to an inflammatory response in the body. This, in turn, overflows into the brain that, by and large, also reflects similar levels of blood sugars as in the body. The brain, starving for energy that it needs to function and think clearly, loses its ability to work in an effective manner. This results in decreased cognitive ability. In the early stages of this process, the pancreas begins to shut down and "wither on the vine," resulting in the need for artificial intake of insulin. In a way, a vital part of the endocrine system, in this case the pancreas, begins to shut down. One can easily see the cascade effects both in the mind and body.

Now let's look at Dr. Hyman's "diabesity," a blended term referring to his insightful way of describing obesity and diabetes and their integrated impact on the body. Although the connection between the two may seem obvious to some people, many people who are overweight or obese have other markers of diabetes in their blood sugar, in many cases untested for years. And it turns out that obesity and fat cells also produce their own brand of inflammatory response, called adipo-cykines. Remember our friends the cytokines, which we discussed in relation to brain inflammation? These are in the same family of inflammatory agents, which the immune system produces as a reaction to an inflammatory response. All of this is an interconnected reaction, where the immune system and inflammatory agents react in a "back and forth" manner with each other. In a sense, the body and immune system are "fighting fire with fire," adding yet *another* layer of inflammatory response. What is the body's response to years of this ever-increasing escalation of inflammatory agents? The answer is what Dr. Hyman calls type 3 diabetes, the third and final aspect of this interconnected "trio" left for us to discuss.

## Type 3 Diabetes

I describe type 3 diabetes as the body being filled with inflammatory agents that can (but not always) overflow into the brain. The blood-brain barrier that is patrolled by our immune system guardians, the monocytes, becomes breached and inflammation increases in the brain. This is apparent, first, as the early stages of Alzheimer's, but increases over time. All of this is a gradual process, sometimes taking decades to come to an obvious conclusion. But there are early warning signs. And it is significant to note that it is estimated that about 25% of all persons 65 or over will develop diabetes.

Although we have discussed to some degree how an unhealthy diet can lead to type 3 diabetes, and how type 3 diabetes connects to Alzheimer's disease, I'll provide here a more detailed description. In summary:

a.   Elevated blood sugar levels, over a period of days, months, years and certainly decades, can become toxic to the body. The source of these elevated blood sugars can come from foods literally higher in sugar content or indirectly through substances such as certain types of more 'modernized' wheat products, found in a great deal of our food products.

b.   These food substances can result in higher insulin resistance in the body.

c.  The first stage of this higher insulin resistance is reflected in what we call pre-diabetes, which can be verified by heightened values in a person's blood tests.

d.  Higher insulin resistance can eventually transition into full-blown diabetes, which is, again, verified by standard blood tests.

e.  'Type 2 diabetes' describes the body's response to insulin resistance, which can result in a failure of the pancreas to create sufficient insulin, requiring additional support (and artificial insulin), as well as regular monitoring to maintain a balance of blood sugar levels and metabolism in the body. Why I believe that 25% of persons age 65 or over develop diabetes is simply a function of time and toxicity. They have had decades' more opportunity to be exposed to toxic levels of sugar, in many forms, and develop an insulin resistance as a result.

f.  The term 'type 3 diabetes' is a way to describe how diabetes creates an insulin resistance in *the brain,* mirroring the insulin resistance in the body. The effect of this is the creation of an inflammatory process in the brain, just as it occurs in the body. One of the consequences of this inflammation in the brain is that the brain cells starve "in the midst of plenty." Type 3 diabetes, then, really indicates a significant connection between the body and the brain.

The "good news" is that not everyone who is older, even with type 2 diabetes, will develop Alzheimer's. The "bad news" is that some *will* develop Alzheimer's (the percentage still to be determined in an ever-aging population). Unfortunately, there is no equivalent of insulin for the brain, as there is in the body. In that sense, even 'treatable' type 2 diabetes in an aging population reflects a higher risk factor for Alzheimer's.

## Heart Disease

There is yet another piece to this puzzle, however, and that is cardiac disease. It turns out that heart disease can be closely related to diabetes. And yes, in a sense, this means it's related to the inflammatory response of the body. Many people who have bypass surgery have undiagnosed diabetes. This was the case with my brother, Roger. I remember quite well when Roger had heart bypass surgery. After the surgery, when visiting him in Arizona, one of the nurses looked at me and said "You'd better get checked out, too."

He had been on heart medication for 10 years and had undiagnosed diabetes during that time. Of course, I ignored her suggestion, but didn't forget the look in her eyes. And after doing all this research, I realized I needed to face the fear that her look sparked. I still wonder what she saw in me that made her say that. Was it genetics, my size, did she see a connection in my physical appearance that she attributed to me being at risk? This research has caused me to take a hard look at myself, which I will tell you more about in Chapter 8.

What I see myself telling you is the story of what I call the "diseases of aging." Although not exclusively the purview of a senior population (for arbitrary reasons I've termed this age 60+), they *are* more commonly found in this population. However, this is also changing.

To help connect diabetes and heart disease to inflammation, there is one more concept to explore: "metabolic syndrome." Metabolic syndrome is a way doctors are beginning to describe the risk factors that, when all are present, lead to increased risk of heart disease. I describe metabolic syndrome as the perfect storm of (to my way of thinking) four different factors, all of which conspire to cause damage or debilitation to the heart:

> High blood pressure
> Diabetes
> Insulin resistance
> Obesity

Since I've already discussed diabetes, insulin resistance and obesity, I'll now target high blood pressure as the final piece of this puzzle. Previously, I mentioned the story of Dr. Upledger and his mentor, Dr. Stacy Howell, who he studied with at the Kirksville College of Osteopathy in the 1960's. Dr. Howell noticed, even then, that inflammation weakens the arterial walls of the heart and vascular system in general, and that cholesterol rushes to try and coat these weakened and thinner tissue areas. At the time, treatment with cholesterol-reducing drugs was just becoming popular, so the inflammatory aspect of vascular damage was lost in the shuffle, so to speak. However, in the last few years researchers have begun to recognize the key role that inflammation plays in the creation of heart disease. As an example, Dr. Mark Houston, an internal medicine specialist from the Vanderbilt University School of Medicine, speaks about heart disease as an auto-immune disease.

In relation to heightened blood pressure, you have a chain of events that begins with arterial and vascular inflammation, which then leads to increased cholesterol coating at the site of injury, followed by greater and greater deposits of cholesterol and artheoroschlerotic plaques. The end result of this is the arteries and veins become clogged and more restricted, ultimately leading to heightened blood pressure. Over time, depending on the amount of damage that occurs, the inevitable cardiac event ensues.

I mention all of this in relation to Alzheimer's because when patients have one or both of the above, their risk of developing dementia and Alzheimer's increases. Common sense tells us when a heart attack or stroke occurs, there is potentially less blood supply to the brain, which then sets the stage for even more impairment of cognitive function.

## Opportunistic Invasion Across the Blood-Brain Barrier:

### Arthritis

Arthritis can certainly be a concern as people age. Since this is related to immune system function, any time you see an "itis" at the end of a word, you can be sure inflammation is at work. A compromised or stressed immune system is less able to regulate and protect itself. In this case targeting the joints and bone, arthritis is also not an uncommon ailment found in dementia patients, yet *another* indication of the inflammatory process at work.

### Osteoporosis

This condition can, of course, be seen in people well before their 60's. Osteoporosis is related to immune system dysfunction, in that when there is an imbalance in bone production, either locally or within the entire body, osteoblasts (which increase bone production) or osteo-clasts (which decrease bone production) are in imbalance. Weakening of the structural support system in our skeletal foundation has at least

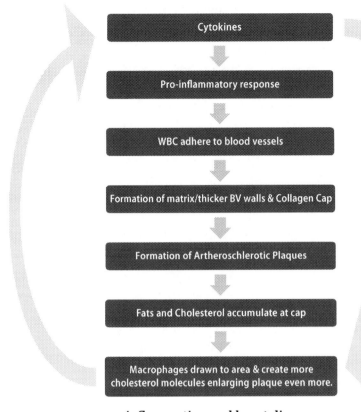

**inflammation and heart disease**

an indirect effect on mobility and flexibility of the body. I'll discuss some suggestions in a later chapter about how to strengthen and balance this system, which is especially important as people age.

**Cancer**

Although not always found in the senior population, the incidence of various types of cancers does show up, not uncommonly, in seniors. There are a couple of factors here that have an influence on long-term health:

1.  *Initial Onset*

    Dr. Upledger used to describe cancer as caused by the disorganization of highly organized cells, which lose their ability to stay properly organized and become simpler, even more embryonic in form. When this occurs, the foundation for tumor formation is laid, like an invading army easily occupying a friendly country. This is a reflection of the immune system's ability and inability to recognize self or non self, resulting in missed cues in the body. Needless to say, there are inflammatory processes at work here, as well. Evidence for this is apparent when even just one of the pro-inflammatory cytokines is at work, namely the tumor necrosis factor or TNF, especially when produced in excess. Unchecked and left in abundance over time, this may, as we have pointed out previously, have an effect on inflammatory processes in the brain.

2.   *Treatment*
Post-chemo and radiation, the immune system must relearn, in a sense, how to function on its own again. The beneficial effects of treatment notwithstanding, any residual toxicity may linger in the body and have some less than charming long-term effects. In point of fact, many patients experience short-term memory disruption and an interruption of cognitive function. Our concern here is any lingering long-term effect in impacting memory and cognition.


## Depression

The distinguished alternative health expert, Dr. Andrew Weil, has described depression as "an inflammatory process." *Depression, too?* It's not a long journey to find the connection between inflammation and depression, even though at first it may not seem obvious. Given an individual who has any or all of the above conditions could be cause for depression, in its own right. However, there is also a physiological connection. When the immune system is dis-regulated, either by inflammatory processes or other invasive factors, brain chemicals in the pituitary, thymus and thalamus act to create factors that affect the emotional structure of the midbrain, and from there, other endocrine systems within the body. Just another reflection of the tip of the iceberg.

Chapter **8**

# What Causes Inflammation?

## Factors or Agents That Cause Inflammation

Many people only think of inflammation when they are referring to a specific injury, say to a muscle. They might take an anti-inflammatory to help reduce the inflammation and ease pain. In essence, these anti-inflammatory drugs or agents are encouraging the immune system to dial back its response to a perceived threat. Many times, however, other parts of the immune system and related organs, such as the liver, spleen or pancreas, are suppressed to achieve the intended results, but this leaves us vulnerable to other infections and diseases. These so-called "possible side effects" are briefly (and usually quite rapidly) mentioned at the conclusion of what often seems like a barrage of TV advertisements for drugs proclaiming they'll "help" people with arthritis, inflamed muscles or other maladies. Pay close attention to the laundry list of potential complications and statements about who should *not* be taking this or that drug, or do whatever research is necessary to determine what's actually safe for you to take.

Interestingly, there are other factors that can cause inflammation throughout the brain and body, which many do not readily associate with inflammation. Remember, it is the immune system in the body that is constantly searching for what is "friend or foe." It has been found that, at least indirectly, substances found in food and the environment can trigger the immune system to defend itself from a perceived threat. What is *not* obvious about this occurrence is that it can build an undesirable immune system response gradually over time *and* cause problems that are both long-term and chronic. It seems appropriate to mention here a few of the key contributors thought to generate inflammation in the brain and body.

## Can Diet and Nutrition Be Involved?

As part of my continuing discovery in this journey, I was somewhat amazed at the influence of nutrition in the creation of inflammation on a long-term basis. Part of this learning took place in my extensive work with autistic children. More often than I expected, the mothers would inform me about how their children would have adverse reactions to various food substances, which indirectly and not so indirectly affected their children's cognitive function and behavior. This alerted me to take a look at this same effect in our senior population, as well, especially when brain function might be affected.

However, I should take a step back and discuss some of the numbers that reflect the large-scale influences of what we consume as a population. Some of these figures I have already mentioned, and some I have not.

If you take into account the number of people estimated to have pre-diabetes (79 million) and add to that the number of diagnosed diabetic patients (28.5 million), roughly one third of the population in the United States is at risk. That's a *substantial* number by anyone's standards.

We've already mentioned Mark Hyman's concept of diabesity. I certainly know the challenge of keeping off weight, or at least until very recently. Many of us have heard through the media or our own reading that carbohydrates and sugars influence weight gain. However, there is another layer to the food story that is not as obvious. Simply put, anything which raises blood glucose levels *beyond* the normal is not good and can lead to problems like weight gain, inflammation and eventually, if unchecked, diabetes. In 2008, the cardiothoracic surgeon and best-selling author Dr. Mehmet Oz appeared on *The Oprah Winfrey Show* and listed five ingredients we need to eliminate or limit in our diet, listed from best to worse: sugar, high-fructose corn syrup (I vividly remember the scene where he poured out this goopy glop), enriched flour (why do they strip flour, and then add some things back in?), saturated fat and hydrogenated oils (also known as trans fats). Dr. Oz cautioned people in his column, "Five Foods That Should Never be in Your Grocery Cart": avoid simple sugars, carbs or unhealthy fats, meats high in nitrates and saturated fats, ingredients you can't pronounce (e.g., thiamine mononitrate or partially hydrogenated soybean oil) "fake" health foods (like certain cookies, yogurt or salad dressings) and canned foods high in sodium.

## The Potentially Adverse Effects of Wheat and Gluten

Yet another factor to pay attention to regarding inflammation is the influence of wheat and wheat-related products. Many foods contain wheat or wheat-related derivatives, sometimes where you wouldn't expect to find them, such as in processed foods. Recently, the potentially negative effects of wheat and gluten have become more widely known and have led to popular gluten-free foods and gluten-free diets. In fact, findings that avoidance of gluten can promote weight loss were recently discussed in the *Journal of Nutritional Biochemistry;* research published in the *Clinical Journal of Gastroentology and Hepatology* linked diarrhea-predominant irritable bowel syndrome (IBS) to gluten and wheat, and a study demonstrating neurological symptoms of autism may be linked to gluten consumption appeared in *Nutritional Neuroscience.*

Interestingly enough, I knew about the benefits of a gluten-free diet long before this became mainstream, because for the last 20 years I've worked on children with various conditions in a therapeutic environment. I've learned most of what I know related to the dysfunction of autism from talking with the mothers of autistic children who are the real "in the trenches researchers" in this area of pediatric medicine. What many of these mothers discovered long ago is that, at least in certain cases, removing gluten from their children's diet improved behavior, and reduced both allergies and other immune system-related symptoms. By trial and error, they learned that gluten can cause an inflammatory response in the body, which in turns influences the immune system. In these highly sensitive children, such an inflammatory response can cause what presents itself much like a tidal wave effect of good and bad.

The key point here is that gluten, which is found in wheat, can cause a rise in blood sugar, high concentrations of which become toxic to the body, and promotes insulin resistance. This, in turn, can cause an inflammatory response in the body. Weight gain may also result from the intake of wheat, which can create its own inflammatory response. Talk about a double blow to the body. By the way, this kind of response also makes it harder to lose weight. Dr. William Davis does a great job of explaining the wheat story in his book, *Wheat Belly.* Dr. Davis, a preventative cardiologist, points out that wheat has evolved from an innocent ancient grain to an industrialized hybrid that exponentially increased yield, solving much of the world's hunger problem. However, in the last 50 years, some side effects have been identified, such as the fact that this food product is not always easily recognized by the digestive systems of both humans and animals (yes, we are even starting to see animals with gluten sensitivities). Dr. Davis points out that eating two slices of bread can raise your blood sugar higher than two tablespoons of pure sugar does!

Something has fundamentally changed, and this something lies in the way this industrialized hybrid of wheat has been bred (no pun intended) and developed. Simply put, the genetics of the vast majority of modern wheat represents a different strain of wheat than the ancient grain our bodies could metabolize easily—that is, without causing harm to itself and without the experience of unwanted side effects. This change in the genetic structure of wheat has affected the health of countless people. As Dr. Davis also points out, when you look at a picture of your parents or grandparents, the vast majority of them had 32-inch waists or wore size 4 dresses. Again, clearly "something" has changed the biochemical and metabolic balance in the body in the past 50 years, and he says this is an indicator of the effects of industrialized or processed foods. I have a hunch these effects have a lot to do with explaining the current "silent" diabetes epidemic in the US.

Another contributor to this subject of nutrition's potentially detrimental influences on the human physiology is Dr. David Perlmutter, whose recent book, *Grain Brain,* ties together the relationship between wheat, carbs and sugar, and the effect these substances have on brain functioning. In his book, Dr. Perlmutter shows how all of the factors we have previously discussed can lead to Alzheimer's and dementia. In essence, he concludes that carbohydrates, gluten and sugars can have a highly toxic effect on the body and lead to a wide variety of autoimmune diseases and Alzheimer's and dementia.

## Genetically Engineered Foods—GMOs: Adding Insult to Injury

There is yet another piece to add to this dismaying "food puzzle"— which I not-so-jokingly say is "adding insult to injury." What I mean by this is that over the last 20–30 years, industrial food giants such as Monsanto have aggressively promoted the use of genetically engineered organisms, or GMOs, into our food supply. My friend, Jeffrey M. Smith, founder of the Institute for Responsible Technology, has brought to light some of the hidden dangers of GMOs, through both feature-length films (*Genetic Roulette: The Gamble of Our Lives*) and books (especially, *Seeds of Deception: Exposing Industry and Government Lies about the Safety of the Genetically Engineered Foods You're Eating*). In simple terms, he explains that DNA has natural ways to protect itself against invasion from other species. This means that to create a GMO requires a way to literally *force* DNA from one organism to another. They do this by infecting the organism with viruses or bacteria to create new DNA, coating the original DNA with tiny metal pellets and firing it into the cells, injecting new DNA into fertilized eggs, or using electric shock to breach the membrane of sperm and forcing new DNA into it. Now, if *that* doesn't sound scary enough, here is a list of actual experiments that have been conducted in the name of developing GMOs (cited on his website: *www.responsibletechnology.org*):

It is now possible for plants to be engineered with genes taken from bacteria, viruses, insects, animals or even humans. Scientists have worked on some interesting combinations:

- Spider genes were inserted into goat DNA, in hopes that the goat milk would contain spider web protein for use in bulletproof vests.

- Cow genes turned pigskins into cowhides.
- Jellyfish genes lit up pigs' noses in the dark.
- Arctic fish genes gave tomatoes and strawberries tolerance to frost.
- Potatoes that glowed in the dark when they needed watering.
- Human genes were inserted into corn to produce spermicide.

Current field trials include:

- Corn engineered with human genes (Dow)
- Sugarcane engineered with human genes (Hawaii Agriculture Research Center)
- Corn engineered with jellyfish genes (Stanford University)
- Tobacco engineered with lettuce genes (University of Hawaii)
- Rice engineered with human genes (Applied Phytologics)
- Corn engineered with hepatitis virus genes (Prodigene)"

Yes, the *idea* is to create something better, and with the food industry in mind, their "inventions" (i.e., GMO foods) will increase food production.

Mr. Smith, however, in following through with penetrating analysis and study, brings up some rather sobering points.

> *"Although there are attempts to increase nutritional benefits or productivity, the two main traits that have been added to date are herbicide tolerance and the ability of the plant to produce its own pesticide. These results have no health benefit, only economic benefit. Herbicide tolerance lets the farmer spray weed-killer directly on the crop without killing it. Crops such as Bt cotton produce pesticides inside the plant. This kills or deters insects, saving the farmer from having to spray pesticides. The plants themselves are toxic, and not just to insects. Farmers in India, who let their sheep graze on Bt cotton plants after the harvest, saw thousands of sheep die! In the case of corn or cotton, genetic engineers have introduced the production of a substance called Bt toxin into the genome of a corn seed. This Bt toxin is highly toxic in its own right, and the idea is that if an insect tries to nibble on the corn, the Bt toxin has the effect of rupturing the intestinal wall of the insect, thereby killing it."*

To paraphrase his conclusion, he acknowledges this GMO "approach" is pretty clever, really. No outside insecticide or spraying needed, as if the seeds were already sprayed with chemical. *However,* there have proven to be some troubling side effects. As noted above, animals that eat the Bt/GMO corn have displayed increased immune system problems, infertility, and weakened intestinal walls. Interestingly, when the farmers take the animals off the GMO corn, the problems seem to disappear. Monsanto scientists insist that this corn, when eaten by animals and then the animals are eaten by humans, is completely safe. However, if these genetically altered traits pass up the food chain, humans run the risk of becoming "Bt toxin factories," as their gastrointestinal (GI) tract manufactures this same substance.

# GMOs and the Inflammatory Process

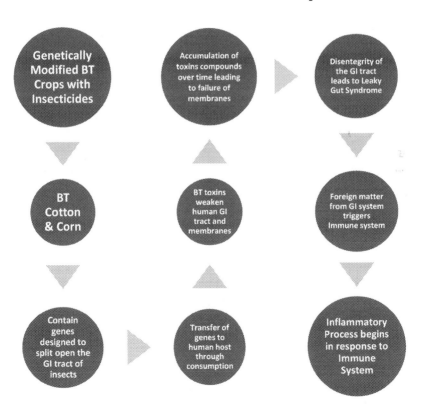

This linkage has actually been shown to exist—that is, in a 2011 study (published in the journal, *Reproductive Toxicology*), doctors at Sherbrooke University Hospital in Quebec found the GMO corn's Bt-toxin in the blood of pregnant women and their babies, as well as in non-pregnant women. (Specifically, the toxin was identified in 93% of 30 pregnant women, 80% of umbilical blood in their babies, and 67% of 39 non-pregnant women.)

Ultimately, people eating GMO corn may suffer a weakened GI tract, due to its having to process genetically modified/toxified corn, which can develop into "leaky gut syndrome," which in turn requires the immune system to help in the digestion of unprocessed food substances that it reads as "foreign substances."

As we know, when the immune system reacts in this way, very often an inflammatory response ensues. Piled high on top of the reaction to other processed foods, such as wheat, most of us need these GMO effects like we need the proverbial hole in the head.

## Stress

Besides noting the effects of nutrition and GMOs, it's interesting to see what researchers have to say about the effects of "stress" from a body-brain chemistry point of view. In explaining the factors of insulin resistance, obesity, and high blood pressure, numerous studies (Cohen et al 2012, Sheridan, Godbout, et al 2012, and Black 2002) point out that stress may have something to do with a lack of balance in the body and the inability to bring the body chemistry under control. This is hardly a surprise, given our own personal relationship to stress in this fast-paced society. However, from a physiological level, it's pointed out that the hypothalamic-pituitary-adrenal axis or HPA-axis, can become dysfunctional due to stress, and therefore produce high cortisol (a hormone related to stress levels) in the body, which in turn raises glucose and insulin levels. These increased glucose and insulin levels, as we've previously noted, can have a less than positive effect on brain functioning and cognition. In essence, what this newest round of research shows is the intimate connection between the mind and body. Specifically, we can now see further that inflammation—which starts in the body, triggered by any number of events we could characterize as 'stress,'—begins to exert a long-term and chronic agitation in all systems of the body, eventually 'overflowing,' as it were, into the brain.

As a teacher of meditation for many years, I routinely speak about blood cortisol levels as a measure of stress, and how meditation techniques can lower these levels. As an instructor of craniosacral therapy, I make the same points from a slightly different point of view. Basically, it's clear that stress contributes to raising the inflammatory response in the body.

## Toxins

I mention toxins primarily to acknowledge the existence of chemical and other non-organic agents that are absorbed by the body from our environment. Since we are surrounded by any number of these agents, overexposure, for many people, may lead to problems over time. As an example of how toxins can affect our health, the story of Erin Brockovich (and the movie with the same name) portrays the drama surrounding industrial pollution (chromium, in particular) at a processing plant, which leads to a marked increase in cancer deaths in a small California town. Of course, the existence of the older, lead-based paints is another example of toxins in the environment that can lead to problems in child development (in this case, many states now require, by law, cautions be given to alert renters or new homebuyers of any potential dangers).

Recently in the United States, awareness of the possible dangers of flame-resistant materials in furniture and foam materials has come to light, with new regulations being implemented in the coming year. Citing the persistent efforts by many citizens and organizations to legislate these toxic materials, a 2012 Pulitzer Prize-winning article in the *Chicago Tribune* exposed the industry responsible for making these products for ignoring their harmful chemicals, which do not prevent materials from burning, but *do* expose users to off-gassing and ongoing cancer-causing chemicals.

On a global level, we are also becoming aware of increased levels of mercury in fresh and saltwater fish. Mercury, a heavy metallic substance that, when entering the human food chain, is difficult to eliminate, has been shown to be associated with symptoms ranging from autism to Alzheimer's. This is just a sample list of toxins in our surroundings. The general reaction by the body to these foreign invaders is to combat their intrusion by reacting with an inflammatory response, as a way of defending itself. Researchers hypothesize ongoing introduction of any or all of these substances, over a continuing period of time, can easily overwhelm the body and can initiate and deepen the disease process (Kempuraj, et al., 2010).

## Genetics

It has become somewhat fashionable to talk about genetics when evaluating a person's propensity toward health or illness, especially in the last few years. There is no doubt that what your mother or father (or for that matter, what your grandparents) carried as a health history is important to consider, when studying one's own state of health, including one's predisposition to inflammatory responses (Montesanto, et al., 2012).

However, there is a change in the air regarding how we look at the outcome for ourselves...and this is most clearly seen in the field of epigenetics. Broadly stated, epigenetics is the view that certain genes can be switched on to promote better health and others switched off to lessen detrimental health effects—that is, we can have an influence on the outcome of any genetic 'predisposition' and minimize the negative impact to ourselves over time. By looking more deeply into epigenetics (which we'll do in the coming chapters), we'll see how we may have a far greater ability to positively affect our future, by recognizing and taking advantage of how we can shape our recovery and regain our health.

## Radiation

Finding out about the effects of radiation has been a hobby of mine since I was a teenager, although for years I didn't realize why. But one day, after I started working in the healthcare field, I asked my mom about my early post-birth history. She told me when I was 10 days old, doctors at the hospital where I was born irradiated my thymus, because it was enlarged. Much later, I found out that an enlarged thymus is actually normal in many babies. And still later, I found out from a nurse-midwife this irradiation procedure was fairly common for infants in the late 1940's and early 1950's.

This was my first exposure, so to speak, to the potential effects of radiation and inflammation on the immune system. It may have been just a coincidence, but I grew up with asthma, which persisted throughout my teenage years. My personal research revealed this exposure was likely just enough to suppress some aspects of my immune system, with asthma and other respiratory challenges coming forward as a result.

Naturally, the question arises, "How does radiation become inflammation?" It turns out that ionizing radiation disrupts the cytoplasm of the cells, creating free radicals and, therefore, toxins on a cellular level. An overabundance of these dysfunctional cells leads to rapid and sometimes catastrophic cell die-off, as in the case of severe radiation poisoning. In most cases, we are not exposed to such high levels of radiation, either medically or from the environment. Still, I believe even low levels of radiation over time have a baseline effect on all cultures and all environments. While much of the time the effect is not acknowledged, when I spoke to my students in Russia about Chernobyl or nuclear testing in the Urals, they reported histories of family members from these regions developing various cancers, respiratory problems and disease, and early death. Another example of the deleterious effects of radiation can be found in Tokyo, Japan, where the baseline level of background radiation is purported to be many times higher now than it was 5 years ago, before the catastrophic tsunami and destruction of nuclear facilities on the northeast coast of Japan.

These are examples of just another factor to be aware of that may contribute to one's susceptibility to inflammation and health challenges.

## Vaccinations

Initially, I wasn't going to mention this one, but recently a friend of mine shared some of her immune system challenges that have been with her for most of her life. It turns out that early in her life, she had received a massive dose of vaccination to help offset a potentially serious condition. I am very familiar with this situation, as I have worked with many children who have developed symptoms of autism after one or more key vaccinations in the first six years of their lives. This is not to object to the principle of immunization, but my observation is that in certain situations, especially in children who have had birth challenges or who are more at risk (meaning birth trauma, long or difficult labor, premature birth, toxicity in the mother or fetus, or general lack of vitality in the early months or years of life), their tiny immune systems may be overloaded, depending on the quantity and timing of these procedures. If you are interested in finding out more about this particular subject, take a look at Dr. Stephanie Cave's book, *What Your Doctor May Not Tell You About Children's Vaccinations* and *Evidence of Harm: Mercury in Vaccines and the Autism Epidemic: A Medical Controversy* by David Kirby.

Now, you may ask, "How does this list of different elements relate to Alzheimer's and dementia?" Primarily, it's a way of pointing out how early health challenges may affect a person's future, by way of setting the stage for an immune system that can become dysfunctional in its regulation and unable to fend for itself over time. (For a comprehensive review of how diet, pharmaceutical intervention and biochemical imbalances can contribute to autism, take a look at Tami Goldstein's book, *Coming Through the Fog.*) It is certainly worth noting that a compromised immune system, whatever the cause, could then lead to the acceleration of the aging process and some of the attendant problems that can go with it.

However, I want to emphatically state there *are* ways to help clear a person's immune system from these effects. In the past, and often still today, the first line of defense is to use medication. In this case, I mean pharmaceuticals, not other types. Unfortunately, it has been found that multiple administrations of certain drugs *can* lead to complications in how the body reacts and how it balances its homeostatic mechanisms, even leading to potential organ damage (or worse), if not closely monitored.

Before we proceed to the next chapter and cover *other* ways for the body to address the effects of the aging process and related dysfunction, as well as how the body heals, let's first discuss a little more about inflammation.

**5 Million:**
**Alzheimer's and Dementia**

**20 Million:**
**Cardiovascular Disease**

**20–100 Million:**
**Diabetes and Pre-diabetes**

**200–250 Million:**
**Diet and pre-existing condition**

## The Pyramid of Inflammation

### Other Contributors to Inflammation

Besides the rather impressive list of inflammation agents we've just gone over, there are other factors that deserve mention. Among these are:

### Infection

As most people know experience, even an innocent scrape or unresolved blister can result in inflammation. Bed sores (decubitus ulcers) can happen to those who are immobile (for even a few days, let alone weeks or months, as in the case of many seniors), which can become infected and then lead to inflammation, even becoming life-threatening in advanced cases. Reasonably so, the immune system is reacting to protect itself; but the overreaction can create an inflammatory response with serious consequences, if left unattended.

**Allergies**

Common allergies are yet another example of how inflammation is a byproduct of the immune system's overresponse. We've all seen flushed or reddened noses, faces and skin that result from an over response called an allergic reaction. As a compliment to our discussion on diet and foods, there is a growing epidemic of food sensitivities than can trigger inflammatory and autoimmune disorders and a dysfunction in the regulation of the gastrointestinal/immune system.

**Physical Trauma**

Especially as a response to long-term injury, those pro-inflammatory cytokines we previously discussed can create an ongoing response that results in either a low-grade or an enhanced inflammation in the body.

**Nutrition Deficiencies**

Interestingly enough, people who look well and healthy *can* suffer from nutritional deficiencies. Even though the body is constantly striving to achieve balance and homeostasis, a lack of iron, calcium, Vitamin D or any number of elements necessary to promote healthy metabolism, digestion or immune system balance *can* cause an inflammatory response (especially when such an imbalance occurs over an extended period of time), This in turn, can create a cascade of effects that will weaken the body, and possibly even the brain and cognitive function. Knowing this, it's easy to appreciate the need for a non-inflammatory diet, especially in an aging population. Clearly, it's also important to correct and heal any imbalances that a diet deficient in one or more essential elements has created over time. In Chapter 11, we'll discuss how to correct and heal such imbalances as I lay out my proposal to reverse Alzheimer's and dementia.

**Autoimmunity**

Many reactions of the immune system can result in an autoimmune response. Conditions such as rheumatoid arthritis, multiple sclerosis, lupus, celiac disease, certain types of cardiac dysfunction, diabetes Type 1, narcolepsy, Hashimoto's thyroiditis, psoriasis, and even the advanced stages of Alzheimer's can all be characterized as an autoimmune response (and this is a very partial list). We've already discussed the role of both the innate and adaptive immune system in relation to brain inflammation. In both inflammatory and autoimmune diseases, aberrant reactions of both these immune system elements can result in the immune system being activated against its own proteins.

## Sedentary Lifestyle

Not moving sufficiently can create inflammation. It is well known that exercise and active lifestyles can decrease inflammation and also reduce the risk of Alzheimer's and dementia. I'll touch again on the importance of exercise (and programs for seniors) in upcoming chapters.

## Lack of Meaning and Purpose in Life

This may seem a bit more abstract, but the loss of meaning and sense of purpose in life can have an adverse effect on health and wellness. Studies derived from the work of David Buettner, a researcher, *National Geographic* explorer and Emmy Award-winning TV producer, show that in communities where shared values and meaning in life are strong, people live longer and better. I'll discuss more about this in Chapter 9.

## Lack of Connection

Although "lack of connection" may be somewhat of an abstract concept, humans seem to thrive on connection with each other. The extensive research studies of Dr. Brene Brown, a professor at the University of Houston's Graduate School of Social Work, have shown that lack of the human connection—the ability to empathize, belong and love—can lead to stress, anxiety and a change in body and brain chemistry, which can result in inflammation.

So we've seen, perhaps to our surprise, that inflammation can be induced by the following:

- Diet and nutrition, including wheat and gluten
- Genetically Modified Foods (GMOs)
- Stress
- Toxins
- Genetics
- Radiation

- Vaccinations
- Infection
- Allergies
- Physical Trauma
- Nutritional deficiencies
- Autoimmunity
- Sedentary lifestyle
- Lack of meaning and purpose in life
- Lack of connection

## Chapter 9

# Going Against the Grain

In discussing concepts like aging and how we heal, and more specifically, whether it's possible to remain well and healthy, especially as we age, I realize not everyone is in agreement about such a possibility. That's why I call this chapter, "Going Against the Grain."

Consider this: in ancient cultures, such as the Vedic culture in India (ca. 2,000–500 B.C.), physicians were paid on the basis of keeping the patient well. If the patient fell ill, the physician was not paid. Imagine what our healthcare system would be like if this were the model? Put in more contemporary terms, the healthcare model would no doubt emphasize prevention, rather than acute care and treatment. Fortunately, there is a change in the air and many more healthcare professionals *are* beginning to consider prevention medicine as a real possibility. As an indication of this change in other countries, doctors in Japan are actually being rewarded and given incentives for keeping their patients well and healthy.

However, we are still at the early stages of this fundamental change. I think it will be good, now, to review some of the current thinking in our society regarding aging, healing and wellness, so we can better address how, when and why the techniques of craniosacral therapy and other adjunctive techniques can be considered as viable options for treatment of Alzheimer's.

As I mentioned earlier, I teach a 4-day class called, "CranioSacral Therapy for Longevity: Reversal of the Aging Process." This is a class for advanced practitioners of CST. However, as these practitioners come from various backgrounds, cultures and beliefs, I feel their views represent a wide spectrum of the population. Please read the statements below about aging, healing and well-being, which were compiled from the attendees. Then, we'll look at how the current culture either supports or does not support these beliefs.

- It's okay to age, as long as I am well and healthy. However, I'm not excited about aging if I'm in ill health.

- Once you start to go downhill, that's the end of the story. So enjoy your good health as long as you can.

- Mom died at 69, and I'm now 67, so I have 2 years left before my number is up.

- My age as an elder is different than my chronological age. If someone were to listen to me blindfolded, they might think I'm 90 years old to be so wise; however, I'm 30 years old and pregnant. Is there a value to being an elder and wise beyond your years? Indeed, is there a value to being an elder?

- My husband is in a nursing home, because it's difficult for him to move easily in and out of bed. Otherwise, I could take care of him. He gets 3 meals a day and minimal support therapies, because we make just enough to not qualify for Medicaid. It's costing us $6,000 a month. I wish more was available for him. I wish something was different.

- Ten-year-old daughter to her mom, working at an Alzheimer's unit" "Mom, why do all these people look dead?"

- I will live to be 120 and I will age well.

- Why don't we ever address the concept of dying? How would our parents feel if we did?

- When I got in and looked at the medications my dad was on, and started to work with the doctors to change some overlapping and conflicting meds, all of a sudden he could speak and carry on a conversation. Dad was better.

- No one is interested in prevention. They wait until there is a crisis, and then insurance (sometimes) covers it.

- I am not defined by my chronological age. I am only as old as I feel.

- We are defined in this culture by how active we are. How many times have we heard, "He is 90 years old and still driving." Or, "She is 85 and still walks 5 miles a day." If we are not active, we are not seen as useful, and therefore elderly.

- Old age is a blessing. People come to me and want to listen.

- I am older than I ever intended to be.

- We are totally unprepared to be parents of our parents. Our parents are dying of different things than before.

- We set our intention for our aging parents; yet at the same time, we see that we need those prayers from the older generations, as well.

- We begin to age the minute we are born. When we are young, we are more physical. As we age, we can become more emotional and spiritual. Perhaps aging is a compliment to all these spheres of life.

- We don't have to be perfect. We just have to be whole.

- I was so busy participating in my pain, I forgot to participate in my life.

- My whole life journey has been to find the missing pieces of my life.

As you can see, this is quite a range of statements about health, aging, one's self-concept and quality of life.

We'll spend the next couple of chapters looking at what might drive the previous statements, observations and concerns. For now, listed below are some beliefs, structures and current practices that support what I see as the prevalent way of thinking. Some of these are so engrained in our culture that it seems "natural" and just "part of the way life is." However, I am bringing these up because they *may* just have an influence on the individual and collective health of our country and the world.

### 1.  A Culture That Celebrates Youth

Youth is a primary value. Indeed, we have been described as an adolescent culture on many levels, including emotional maturity. In traditional cultures, the elders are seen as a resource for wisdom. They have a place or function in the culture and their counsel is sought after. In contemporary culture, the elders are often separated and "warehoused" or at best isolated from others.

### 2.  Current Medical Model: Medical Specialization

Since the 1790's, when the first medical clinics were established in Europe, medical specialization has gained an inevitable momentum. That's why it's possible to have a cardiac specialist, a GI specialist, a respiratory specialist, an immunologist, a neurologist and a psychiatrist, none of whom typically communicate or speak with each other. This can lead to confusion in treatment, especially with seniors.

### 3.  Current Medical Model: Symptoms, Not Cause

Also in the current medical model, doctors are often experts at diagnosis. However, as reflected in the statement above (#2) on specialization, the evaluation of a patient may focus on a particular symptom and not the underlying cause, if indeed, it is understood. The emphasis on tests, many of which are expensive and sometimes unnecessary, also is emphasized in the current medical model. Once a test offers a validation of some syndrome or disease process, then surgery or drugs are offered as a solution (oftentimes, even when such treatments don't address the primary cause or regularly result in creating lasting improvement).

### 4.  Illness, Not Prevention

When one is chasing symptoms, one is, in a sense, waiting to close the door after the horse has left the barn, clinically speaking. A patient will come in complaining of a symptom or multiple symptoms, on the basis of which, after appropriate (or inappropriate) tests are given, a diagnosis is made, and then recommendations, such as pharmaceutical treatment, are given. One could ask, "Are there any prior conditions or underlying factors that have contributed to this symptom/these symptoms/this illness?" One could further ask, "If these conditions or factors could be identified earlier on, might it prevent the illness in the first place, or at least minimize the impact of the current illness?" This represents the difference between preventative and illness-based medicine. As we will see in the following sections, the current system rewards and recognizes illness-based medicine from an economic and structural point of view. As Dr. Don Berwick, former head of Medicare/ Medicaid put it, "It would well serve us to put the money into health and not illness."

### 5. Economic Incentives: Pharmaceutical Intervention

Pharmaceutical companies have really been around in their modern form for about the last century. Before that, so-called "nature-based" remedies and natural healing methods were more of a standard in the medical community. Indeed, in the late 1800's, there was a widely held belief that within the body existed a "natural pharmacy," which could be recruited to help heal the body. The idea from *many* ancient medical traditions is that the body's "inner intelligence" knows a great deal about how to heal and what to do to cure an illness. As part of this model, the focus on food or nutrition as medicine was part of the belief system.

This is not to discount the role of modern drugs in saving lives and assisting in the healing process, especially in the acute or emergency phase of treatment.

Still, pharmaceutical treatment is now, by and large, based on an industrial system of manufacturing, seemingly well-suited to a mass and sophisticated urban society. Given that it can take hundreds of millions of dollars and years of development to bring a drug to market, it would be wise to recognize the economic and profit incentives that are available with the utilization of prescription allopathic drugs.

As a former entrepreneur and inventor of high-tech solutions for the industrial automation industry, I am well familiar with spread-sheets and how to justify an investment opportunity. "Return on investment" is the mantra of the investment community. Also, one of the basic principles in creating wealth, pointed out by Napoleon Hill and other "creating abundance" business leaders, is that if you have a product that is needed by millions of people and you have a solution, there are fortunes to be made. Even better is a product that is needed on an ongoing basis, ideally monthly, such as rent or a utility, cable or telephone bill. This is known as a cash stream-based industry, and it has its own inherent value. Just ask Henry Ford, John D. Rockefeller, Bill Gates or the CEOs of AT&T or Direct TV.

How does this apply to the pharmaceutical industry? Let's look at some of the numbers. As of 2012, global revenues for the combined pharmaceutical industries was $643 billion. The US accounted for almost half of that, or $289 billion. And looking back, in 1999, 15% of the world's population who lived in high-income countries purchased and consumed about 90% of the total medicines. In other words, those who could afford it the most bought the product. And that is projected to increase. In the next few years, pharmaceutical revenues are expected to exceed $880 billion annually.

How does this relate to a cash-stream industry? Does this fit the criteria? If you do the simple math and divide the total annual revenue by twelve, you get about $24 billion monthly income for the US. That includes all medications consumed by people in the US. Admittedly, not all of this is profit. But as an expected, predictable cash revenue producer, this certainly fits the bill. Even more to the point, a certain percentage of this annual revenue is *recurring.*

There are a couple lines of thought to consider here. Remember, these are ongoing monthly revenues. Put another way, these are return customers. Did you ever think to ask the attending doctor, "How long do I (or my parents) need to be on these drugs?" or "Is this a temporary measure or a permanent solution?" The answer anyone gets, of course, may vary. A reasonable response may be, "Until the symptoms subside" or "Indefinitely," which would not be an uncommon response. One phrase that sticks in my mind comes from a current pharmaceutical commercial on TV, in which the white-jacketed doctor (actually a paid actor) is holding up a mirror to people passing by. The announcer says in a reassuring voice, "When diet and exercise aren't enough." *Why not?* I ask. *Is there an underlying cause that might be overlooked?*

The above "approach" reveals the "drug management-to-goal" type of approach, which sets parameters on acceptable limits for each dysfunction, instead of looking deeper at the root of these issues. Again, the drugs help manage and bring the numbers into balance, but may not bring any long-term solution without ongoing administration of the drug (or alternative drug) in question. Shannon Brownlee, a medical journalist and Acting Director of the New America Foundation Health Policy Program, said on a recent CNN special on US healthcare, "The US healthcare system is not interested in getting you better. Indeed, it just wants to keep you well enough to keep you coming back for more treatment." *And* coming back to spend more money on treatment, which often enough seems to be just about managing or masking symptoms, instead of addressing and resolving them. At least, that's another perspective to consider. *But who could blame the pharmaceutical industry from wanting to make an ongoing profit?*

And while we are on the subject of allopathic medicine and pharmaceutical intervention, I would like to mention an important, but often ignored aspect of both: *side effects.* The nature of allopathic medicine, and the substrates and the biochemical delivery systems it employs, often cause anything from mild to severe side effects. That's why drug commercials often rattle off a laundry list of symptoms you need to be aware of. Or why, when taking a drug, you receive a pamphlet listing studies and percentages of undesirable outcomes. The pharmaceutical companies are legally obligated to do so, and that's why many drug commercials sound as much like a legal disclaimer as a commercial for suggested use (which encourages you to ask your doctor, in any case).

Again, employing common sense, does anyone bother to ask why there are so many side effects for a particular drug? What *causes* the side effects? What organ or molecular mechanism is the drug targeting? Since when has death become merely a side effect? And does anyone truly understand how multiple drugs and multiple side effects interact with each other? These questions are especially important to ask in a senior population, comprised of people who are often more sensitive and vulnerable.

## 6.  Insurance Companies/Senior Care Facilities

This factor, while of obvious concern to all age groups, again holds great importance for senior care, and is somewhat intertwined with how senior living and nursing homes take care of their patients. We have, of course, been recently bombarded with information about the pros and cons of health care and insurance (given passage of the Affordable Care Act), and I only wade into these waters to give you a brief perspective about what *are* currently recognized as viable treatment options and what are *not,* based on discussions with therapists working in senior care facilities.

A student in training who helps Alzheimer's patients recently shared a buzz word with me: "productive time." What that means is how much time during the day a therapist is expected to be productive, that is, how much of their day can be billed to a particular modality by their employer or by referral to Medicare or Medicaid. The magic number, it seems, is 85%. That means that in order to meet corporate projections of productivity, 85% of their time must be related to some billable activity. The therapist in question shared with me that along with her colleagues, she determined that this equation left approximately 13 minutes a day for bathroom breaks, writing notes, or conferring with other coworkers about the condition of a patient.

I bring this up because there are categories that *are* covered for treatment and those that *are not.* It's really a bit more complicated than what I am explaining to you; but in essence, any manual therapy, such as craniosacral therapy, even if it were understood by the insurance company, is not covered. Our competition in the industry is really the time it takes to administer a medication (which may mask a symptom or in the case of Alzheimer's, not have a demonstrable long-term effect): say, 30 seconds, versus the 5–10 minutes a day to administer an easily learned hands-on technique, such as the StillPoint in CST. That is really not a lot of extra time, but in a 100-bed facility, it is employee time that adds up. It may be easier to administer a medication, especially if it is covered by any combination of insurance, Medicare or Medicaid.

In fairness to the senior care industry, most employees, whether they be CNA's (certified nursing assistants), PT's (physical therapists), OT's (occupational therapists) or speech therapists, are usually swamped. These compassionate people can be trained to take an extra five minutes to answer a question, listen compassionately, or fluff a pillow. (By the way, none of those just mentioned fall under billable minutes, hours, or activity.) But being who they are, most of these folks *will* take the time, even if it comes at a cost to them.

There is another dimension to this time-sensitivity issue, one that our study directly addressed: agitation. It's not uncommon for a resident with early- to late-stage Alzheimer's to become agitated during the day. This is actually a time management problem, because CNA's and others do not have the time to listen, calm a patient, and allow them time to get settled, especially as the disease progresses. The solution? Not always, but depending on the facility, drugs such as Adavan or Haladrol (agitating or mood-altering medications, to put it nicely) may be administered. This leaves the patient in a calm and cooperative state. It may also leave them somewhat unresponsive and unaware of their environment. But the agitation problem is solved. We found in our study that a daily 10–15 minute application of a craniosacral StillPoint decreased agitation significantly.

This, of course, brings up the issue of quality of life for the patients in these facilities. Although not intended, there can be a conflict between the time needed to administer to patients in the standard medical model and the time needed to take care of them in a way that puts a premium on their quality of life. However, one factor that may not be taken into account is the indirect costs of *not* attending to these more "humane" and social needs. Many senior care facilities, whether they are assisted living, part-time or full-care nursing, are sensitive to how they are perceived in the category of "quality of life" for the residents. It is usually the children of the parents who drive this sensitivity, and indeed, are ones who may recommend the same facility to other friends and family—that is, for residents fortunate enough to have family somewhere in their area or in their life. If not, the quality of life may fall on state or federally mandated guidelines to look after their long-term care.

Additionally, there is yet another economically driven factor: therapist training. There are actually time and resources set aside for annual continuing education for Alzheimer's in many facilities. Because it takes about two days for the "basic training" in craniosacral technique, this is also a consideration on a facility-wide basis.

In summary, from an insurance and senior healthcare point of view, what we have put forward here is a reflection of the difference between illness-based and preventative medicine. And in this section, there is really no judgment—rather, it is just a reflection of the system as it is currently set up. Many of us would agree there is room for innovation and improvement. Dr. Dean Ornish provides a good example. Dr. Ornish is a pioneer in "heart healthy" medicine. He was bold enough years ago to publish a study, claiming that the effects of heart disease could be cured and even reversed. He created quite a controversy at the time with his research and claims. Over the years, however, his findings were accepted and integrated into cardiac treatment and thinking. Because his approach was also strongly "preventative," it took some additional time to be accepted. Indeed, it took 16 years for Medicare to approve his "heart healthy" lifestyle program. As Dr. Ornish shared in a recent interview, "When we change reimbursement, we change the system."

## 7. Genetics

Genetics has been a popular subject in the area of medical evaluation over the last decade or two. As part of the evaluation and health history of a patient, it is somewhat routine to ask what diseases a relative or parent may have had. This seems like common sense; but especially in instances where no other factors seem to be at cause, genetics can become the default diagnosis. The concept of a genetic predisposition in a family toward a particular disease stems also from this thinking. So it is reasonable for a patient to think, "Well, if Mom or Dad had heart disease (or cancer or Alzheimer's), will I get it too?"

If the prevalent medical model were purely preventative in nature, this type of thinking might be useful. However, many patients, holding firmly to their belief systems, might see genetics as a "sentence," rather than just useful information. Indeed, there have been some science fiction movies where, perhaps in an exaggerated fashion, one's entire career and station in life are predetermined by their blood chemistry, DNA and related analyses—a "brave new world," where science and technology pre-judge the fate of civilization.

However, more recently, a new way of thinking about genetics has emerged that we touched on in the previous chapter: the field known as epigenetics. Simply put, epigenetics says that we may be able to influence genetic outcomes through nutrition and other means. In effect, we can switch *off* the genes that may be harmful to us and switch on the genes that support the best health. Genetically speaking, we are, in a sense, stacking the cards in our favor. Of course, in the realm of craniosacral therapy, this fits in with our view of using subtle intention and dialogue to create a positive change in a patient's future.

## 8. Time

"I'm late, I'm late for a very important date!" says the rabbit in Lewis Carroll's *Alice in Wonderland*. Carroll was, in effect, not just a writer, but also a mathematician, long before Einstein understood that time was relative. In other words, how we perceive the passage of time or the quality of time influences how fast or slow it is perceived. In this case, genetics and time are intertwined, because time represents where we came from, and indeed influences the outcome of where we are going. This, of course, also references epigenetics and the belief that we can turn on and off the genes that may have a detrimental or beneficial effect on our health. So, our belief about time can also, in a sense, shape the outcome of our well-being. Consider the statements, "I'm running out of time" or "Time is against me." On the other hand, also consider the attitude, "Time is on my side."

## Blue Zones

As an overall support for maintaining a healthy diet, nutrition and lifestyle as we age, I wanted to mention the concept of 'Blue Zones.'

I recently found out that the state of Iowa has initiated a program as part of its goal to become the healthiest state in the nation by 2016. Select communities are participating in a "transformation process" and becoming Blue Zones Communities, where people live longer and better.

Here is an excerpt from the Blue Zone website (*www.bluezones.com*):

> "In 2004, Dan Buettner teamed up with National Geographic and hired the world's best longevity researchers to identify pockets around the world where people lived measurably better. In these Blue Zones, they found that people reach age 100 at rates 10 times greater than in the United States. They found the extra 10 years that we're missing.
>
> After identifying the world's Blue Zones, Buettner and National Geographic took teams of scientists to each location to identify lifestyle characteristics that might explain longevity. They found that the lifestyles of all Blue Zones residents shared nine specific characteristics. We call this list of characteristics 'The Power 9.'"

I'm not going to go into detail regarding all nine characteristics, but here is a list of them. Feel free to check out the website, if you would like to read more.

1. Move Naturally
2. Purpose
3. Down Shift
4. 80% Rule—eating to 80% full
5. Plant Slant
6. Wine @ 5
7. Belong to a faith-based community
8. Loved Ones First
9. Right Tribe

*"This is one of the few times in history since Hippocrates that we have not explained the causes of disease to our patients."* —Dr. Dean Ornish

Chapter **10**

# How We Age—An Ounce of Prevention

In the previous chapters, I've pointed out some of the formidable details about Alzheimer's, including its primary symptoms, the nature of brain inflammation, how this same inflammatory process is found in the body, and I've discussed how the food we eat and the lifestyle we lead can cause some of these underlying conditions. I've also shared with you a few of the heartbreaking stories of Alzheimer's and its effects on both seniors and their families. However, now it's time to share some "good news" and look at the message of hope that the natural healing process of the body offers.

Clearly, our culture is changing regarding how we view and approach aging. The MacArthur Research Network on an Aging Society points to an ever growing, healthier population, and the importance of changing public policy to accommodate these facts, and a Pew research article points out globally how this changing view about aging is reflected in the demographics of a number of countries around the world (MacArthur Foundation, 2013, "Growing Older But Not Old: Insight on Aging and Health").

In the following couple of chapters, I'll be discussing the somewhat radical concepts of prevention and reversal of—and even regeneration from—the effects of disease, *even* those maladies that affect the brain (e.g., Alzheimer's and dementia). In doing so, I'll hopefully be pointing the way for readers and the medical community to recognize the huge potential benefits of the BodyEnergy Longevity Prescription, especially in its support of the senior population and those who are nearing that age of life.

In the course of any discussion of what it means to age (especially into one's senior years), a legitimate question arises: "Can a person remain well, healthy and vital as they move into their "golden years," *and also,* at the same time, actually gain wisdom?" Dr. Bill Thomas calls this, "transitioning into 'elderhood.'"

I believe that elderhood, as a part of the aging process, involves the process of gaining a certain balance and emotional maturity. Just as bringing up the concept of diet and nutrition may be difficult for some, in the same manner being in touch with our inner feelings and emotions may raise some challenges. Yet it is my consistent experience in practicing craniosacral therapy that those who have more emotional access, connection and completion in their lives remain healthier, happier and younger. Remaining healthy as we age, then, is not merely an extension of physical reserve. I maintain it also involves continuing in the process of emotional and spiritual growth. Perhaps this insight is one "gift" those of us who face the issue of aging have to offer the younger generation.

Having said all of this, let's look at the traditional measures of the 'normal' aging process.

The subject of aging is a sensitive one. Simply bringing it up in conversation can raise subtle, yet challenging issues and force people to confront their belief systems and the various prevailing systems of thought. Still, I'd like to share with you, now, three different ways of looking at the aging process:

## 1. "Young Old" and "Old Old"

Clinical psychologist Mary Pipher has written a wonderful book entitled, *Another Country: Navigating the Emotional Terrain of Our Elders,* in which she distinguishes a psychological divide between the older and younger generations *and* coins the concept of "young old" and "old old." What she means by this is that anyone who is past a certain age—say, 60 and older (I myself being in this category)—*can* actually fall into the category of "young old." That is, we are chronologically in a specific age range, but are sufficiently active, healthy, out there in the world, and psychologically in a younger mental frame, so as to "qualify" as being "young old." For many of us in the Baby Boomer generation, the qualities ascribed to this label fit the framework we wish to embrace.

Dr. Pipher's other distinct category is "old old." These are people in the same age range who, for whatever reason, appear to be more severely limited in their mobility, overall physical health and mental capacity. She points out that after certain crises or occurrences in life, the characteristics of "old old" become predominant. The distinction she makes here can be of crucial importance, so I will later address how even this stage of aging may be reversible. In summary, Dr. Pipher's concept of "young old" and "old old" is one way of looking at the way we define the aging process.

## 2.  Chronological and Biological Age

This is a distinction I began actively using as I started teaching my class, "CranioSacral Therapy for Longevity: Reversal of the Aging Process." The idea is simply that "chronological age" means your "official" documented age, or your passport age, as my Russian friends like to put it. "Biological age," on the other hand, is an indicator of the "wear and tear" that has accumulated in your body over time. Biological age is a bit subjective to determine, although there are scientific measures such as lung capacity, muscle strength, cognitive abilities and overall stamina, which are reflective of one's biological age. All of us have known people who look a lot younger than they appear, and we are surprised to find out they are chronologically older. On the other hand, we've all observed folks who appear a lot older than they look. It reminds me of the title of a 1960's song by Duane Eddy, called "Forty Miles of Bad Road." Then there are some people (probably the majority) who look just about even: the biological and chronological ages seem the same.

What is the value in knowing the difference? In a sense, the amount of "buffer" we have between biological and chronological age tells us how well we are aging. If someone, for instance, is chronologically 60, but biologically 50, then they have ten years of buffer to work with. That means, the probability is higher that they have more physiological reserves to draw on when the body faces a crisis, and will likely live longer and better, in most cases. Remember the example in the last chapter, where one of my students said, "Mom lived till 69 and I'm 67, so I have 2 years left till my number is up?" Do you think it would make a difference for her to know her "biological age"?

Perhaps she is actually biologically 58, and not 67? And what if her biological age could be extended as she ages? This example also illustrates how the predictions of genetics can be modified. What if her inner wisdom possessed and was able to work with that important information? Taking this a step further, what if she had more resources with which to actually initiate change *and* the confidence drawn from knowing that positive change is possible? Acknowledging the potential positive effects of knowing one's biological age may not be easy for some, but consider this: making use of this knowledge may have a significant influence on a person's quality of life and how we age.

On the other hand, what if one's biological age is more than one's chronological age? That is, what if a 60-year-old, chronologically speaking, is biologically 10 years older? Then, this person would most probably fall into the category of the "old old." Certainly, this situation *could* arise in instances of trauma or other conditions that affect the body negatively. However, some pertinent questions one might ask here include: Is this person destined to have a negative 10-year age gap? In other words, is aging a one-way street? Can we address this person's condition and if so, how? That is, can the gap between biological and chronological age be narrowed? How would this effect the quality of one's life? Obviously, these are important questions and we'll focus in on them in greater detail shortly.

### 3.  Normal and Pathological Aging

I leave until last the most traditional distinctions, those being between normal and pathological aging. In the past decade or so, many universities around the country have developed departments of gerontology, which is a reflection, I think, of our aging population. These institutions have standardized definitions for and theories about the aging process, which are currently used in the field and which I'll be briefly reviewing below.

## Normal Aging

Per traditional definitions, the standard biological theories about normal aging include the following:

*Cellular Aging*—The idea here is that aging is programmed and limited, due to the number of cells that are produced, and the presumed biological limit to a lifespan. In a very real sense, the cells wear out just like the parts of a car wear out. (Remember, this is a theory, but it has been around for a while.)

*Random Damage*—Although this term makes me chuckle (reminding me of having to talk to an insurance adjuster), the concept here is that, as the name implies, normal wear and tear affect the body and the aging process. Referencing our previous discussion, such wear and tear would affect biological age in an adverse way.

*Cross Linkage*—While sounding a bit more technical, cross linkage refers to the concept that protein fibers making up the connective tissue holding us together lose elasticity. Simply put, we become less flexible and increasingly stiffer. Think of aging, here, as less fluid flow and greater dryness...which brings to mind a passage written by William Shakespeare:

> *The sixth age shifts*
> *Into the lean and slipper'd pantaloon,*
> *With spectacles on nose, and pouch on side,*
> *His youthful hose well sav'd, a world too wide,*
> *For his shrunk shank, and his big manly voice,*
> *Turning again towards childish treble, pipes*
> *And whistles in his sound.*

*Homeostatic Imbalance and Allostatic Load*—Simply put, these terms put together convey the idea that it takes us longer to recover from stress and stressful events as we age. We are all familiar with the concept of homeostatis, or how well the body maintains balance even in a chaotic and disorganized environment. That's what homeostatic balance or imbalance refers to. Yet that term in and of itself did not seem to capture the notion of aging in our culture. Even seniors in their 'golden years' (who make adjustments to maintain homeostatic balance) regularly experience stress, worry or anxiety. In that sense, the more recent concept of "allostatic load" helps to describe how we deal with the faster pace of society, how long it takes to recover from a particular set of circumstances, *and* how circumstances affect our mental and physical balance.

I know from my experience with autistic children just how fragile their psychology can be if there is too much input too quickly. And so it can be as we age, *if* we lose the flexibility of our nervous system. From a psychological point of view, as we get older, we *can* become less flexible and more cautious in our view of the world, and even new ideas. After all, if it takes us longer to recover from stressors and stress, why put ourselves in the position of *anything* that might cause additional stress to us, either mentally or physically?

Again, the above list represents the commonly accepted theories of "normal aging." As I've mentioned, depending on how we take care of ourselves, the outcomes of normal aging can vary greatly. In a future chapter, when I talk about resources, I will point out how we can "hold the line," so to speak, and optimize our health, well-being, and quality of life. In the context of Dr. Pipher's concept of "old old" and "young old," many of you readers may fall into the latter category. However, there are practices we can adopt to challenge even the traditional concepts of cellular aging, random damage (even if it has occurred), cross linkage (alternative techniques, such as craniosacral therapy and meditation, can enliven and promote elasticity on a cellular level), and, of course, allostatic load (by promoting greater endocrine system balance with a variety of techniques).

Normal aging is easier than pathological aging to address—in terms of slowing, halting or reversing it—simply because, as the saying goes, "An ounce of prevention is worth a pound of cure." Or put another way, reversal of the aging process is easier to address when there has been less trauma to the body. However, having said that, we do have to take seriously the principle of prevention... *and* take more responsibility for our role in the outcome of aging and our quality of life, as time, *our* time, goes by.

## Pathological Aging

Let's now look at "pathological aging," the category of aging into which Alzheimer's and dementia fall. Using Dr. Pipher's terminology and paradigm, this is also the realm of the "old old."

I'll briefly describe below the three key concepts of pathological aging, which are defined as physical changes resulting from disease and are *not* a normal part of the aging process.

*Cellular Mitochondria*—Investigation at the cellular level reveals that mitochondria are sub-cellular components, which are responsible for the generation and transfer of energy in our cells, both locally and throughout the body, thereby giving us the ability to move and accomplish daily and long-term tasks. Remember when we discussed insulin resistance and the inflammatory processes in the body? Insulin resistance is an indication of how *inefficient* the body has become in drawing on the energy to function—both in the mind and in the brain. The inflammatory process, in this sense, indicates how much 'noise' or inefficiency or drag there is on the resources of the body. And so, what if the body is not able to draw upon glucose and other energy derivatives that provide the mitochondria with the resources they need to energize and move the body? What are the short- and long-term effects of this on the cells, organs and other systems of the body? Well, the effects are reflected in the development of pre-diabetes and diabetes, for one, which can show up as a strain and degradation in the liver, pancreas and/or kidneys. And this is why cellular mitochondria are so important. In a sense, improperly functioning cellular mitochondria are like having an economic meltdown on a body-wide level. The bottom line is, current research indicates that mitochondrial problems can show up as a metabolic dysfunction, which in turn accelerates the aging process (Hotamisligil, G.S., *Nature* 14 December 2006).

*Inflammatory Mechanisms*—We've discussed inflammatory mechanisms extensively already, but the essential point to grasp here is this: reversal of the negative effects of inflammatory processes, both in the brain and body, is where we can find the greatest hope for addressing pathological aging. When we look at all three of these factors together (i.e., cellular mitochondria, inflammatory mechanisms, and the teleomere/telomerase axis), we can see just how interrelated they are.

*Telomere/telomerase axis (DNA)*—This is one of the newer and more cutting edge ways of describing pathological aging. Think of telomeres as the "end caps" of the strands of DNA (or like the plastic ends that surround our shoelaces). When these end caps become unraveled, the DNA that is replicated in our body throughout our lifetime can begin to reproduce itself in a less than faithful copy. If you've ever used a photocopier and have made copies of a copy, you will see that the images are not as crisp as the original.

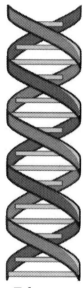

**Telomere**

Just like that, the result is inaccurate or incomplete reproduction of those very cells we have discussed, which are necessary to maintain full and complete functioning as the body ages. Dr. Elizabeth Blackburn won the Nobel Prize in medicine in 2009 for her work in identifying the mechanisms that reveal how these telomeres behave. In her words, "As telomeres get shorter, life gets shorter."

The concept of normal aging presents the possibility of living a long and healthy life. In the last chapter, "Going Against the Grain," we discussed some of the prevailing attitudes about what is and what isn't possible as we increase our chronological age. What if we could stack the cards in our favor as our lives went on? What if "the third act" of our lives could be our best act ever? Is it possible to really take care of ourselves to prevent the more dire consequences of pathological aging?

Our current healthcare system has been set to reimburse acute or chronic conditions, which often demand expensive treatments and medications. This is where the direction of change in current healthcare, insurance and government Medicare and Medicaid is moving, perhaps slowly, toward a tipping point. I believe it is inevitable, as economic pressures mount with an aging population, that at some point, both economic and political interests will arrive at the same conclusion: "prevention" saves vast amounts of resources and eliminates the economic pressure on younger generations.

I call upon you, the reader, to become more educated about how prevention creates value both for yourselves and your family. Here I am suggesting that the concept of preventative maintenance can become a part of every person's daily life. I'll discuss this in greater depth in the following chapters.

## 10 Steps for Prevention.

Let me leave you with a few "action steps," which are my best suggestions to reinforce the concept of prevention:

**1: Diet and Nutrition:** This, of course, is a big subject. As we've discussed, what we eat and how we eat can have a significant influence on our short- and long-term health. One doesn't need to go 'whole hog,' so to speak, to effect positive change. Even a few changes in the intake of sugars and carbohydrates can have a significant and positive effect on our ability to think, be active, and age more gracefully. There are many resources to help get informed about this, and I'll mention just a few: Dr. Mark Hyman's *Blood Sugar Solution,* complete with quizzes about your 'inflammatory index' and some nice suggestions for healthy, tasty food. In the same vein is Dr. David Perlmutter's *Grain Brain: The Surprising Truth about Wheat, Carbs, and Sugar—Your Brain's Silent Killers,* which also explores the relationship between food and mental functioning, and also has suggestions on how to prepare healthy, tasty food. (Notice I use the work tasty. In my own experience, if something tastes good, a change of 'diet' does not seem like a punishment, but more of a way to enjoy food and feel better as well.) I would also suggest taking a look at Drs. Marwan Sabbagh and MacMillan's *The Alzheimer's Prevention Cookbook,* which provides a good background on the relationship between food and Alzheimer's, as well as some great healthy food suggestions and recipes. In our upcoming chapter on resources, we'll touch on this subject, as well.

**2: Exercise.** It seems intuitive that 'just moving' is good for the body and overall general health. Again, even beginning with small steps can make a big difference. If one needs "official confirmation" of this, studies show that C-reactive protein, associated with stress, hypertension and inflammation, are all reduced by exercise (Ford, E.S. 2002). Walking just 20–30 minutes a day can significantly reduce the risk of Alzheimer's. For those whose mobility are challenged or may be a bit older, there are other alternatives, as well, such as tai chi for seniors, and exercise programs that can even be practiced in a wheelchair. I was recently inspired to see a documentary on war vets who have a stringent work out routine and keep in great physical and psychological shape. Exercising with friends can also reinforce doing regular exercise. (And yes, if you must, you can always have your cell phone with you!)

**3: Blue Zones and the Power of Nine.** I've mentioned in a previous chapter. This is Dan Buetlner's Blue Zone concept, in which he studied the nine key practices of seniors around the world who age the longest and have the best quality of life. Take a look at *http://www.bluezones.com* for more information. One of my favorite recommendations from the Power of Nine is *wine at 5*, where seniors in select communities regularly enjoy a social glass of wine in the later afternoon hours.

**4: CranioSacral Therapy.** I've spent a good deal of time pointing our how craniosacral therapy (or CST) can help combat and reduce brain inflammation and the beginning stages of Alzheimer's. This is because CST encourages the flow of cerebral spinal fluid or CSF, and thereby helps support overall brain health. Put simply, the more fluid flow the better. Besides initial studies on the effectiveness of CST on aging and brain health, we are adding daily to our case history studies from therapists around the country.

There are a couple of ways to use CST as a preventative technique:

a. Contact a local 'senior specialist' in CST who can give you a treatment (this usually takes about an hour) and can help develop a plan, based on their assessment, of how frequently it would be useful to take advantage of this relaxing technique.

b. The 'mini-intensive' program offered by the BodyEnergy Institute. We also have available a 3-day mini-intensive program, in which a client can come for two hours at a time, up to 3 days in a row, and have a number of therapists working on him or her at the same time. The mini-intensive program was created because I found that many clients (of all ages) had experienced a lot of trauma in their lives (from car accidents to disease processes and beyond), and so they could benefit from the "intensified" amount of CST work we could provide them in such a setting. This concentrated intensive program has become very popular, and, based on my own experience, it provides a highly effective way to both reduce accumulated 'wear and tear' in the body (recall the cellular aging and random damage concepts discussed above) *and* reverse the aging process. For more information on how to find a craniosacral therapist who specializes in senior care or to learn more about the mini intensive programs I mentioned, you can contact me at *www.BodyEnergy.net* or refer to the Upledger Institute at *www.upledger.com*.

**5: Training in the CranioSacral Therapy Technique.** These 2-day classes for laypeople (no prior experience necessary) provide the knowledge and hands-on instruction in how to perform some simple CST techniques. There are currently two classes being offered: "CranioSacral Therapy for Longevity—Applications for the Treatment of Alzheimer's and Dementia (CSLAD) and "CranioSacral Therapy for Longevity-Applications for Prevention and Healthy Aging (CSLAP)." For a list of available classes, go to *www.BodyEnergy.net*.

**6: Building Community.** Earlier, I mentioned that Baby Boomers (and younger generations, in general) don't necessarily want to age in the same way or manner their parents have. A part of this involves creating a different way of building community. Examples of this are families that are multigenerational (where parents, grandparents and grandchildren all live together in various configurations); spiritual and alternative communities, where shared belief systems are common, independent living is the norm and support is available as needed; or

communal living where there are shared resources (community din-
ing, preventative healthcare) *and* individual residences, as well. We are
seeing the growth of new alternatives not imagined even 10 years ago.
Since this is an ongoing conversation, I invite you to become informed
and part of this "movement" by going to *www.BodyEnergy.net/commu-
nity.* Take a look at the resources there and consider sharing your own
insights and views.

**7: Meditation, Visualization and Yoga.** At a recent visit to a senior
community, I was again reminded of how much seniors can worry and
display anxiety. Not everyone, to be sure, but it is not an uncommon
complaint to hear, "It's hard to relax and settle down." Of course, those
of us who are younger may have the same concerns. There are some
proven techniques that can assist in the reduction of stress. Yoga (at
least the type that teaches gentle stretching and easy movement) can
be a great ally for the reduction of stress. Kripalu Yoga center on the
East coast is a great resource for learning about yoga, as well as any
number of resources on the internet. You can contact Kripalu or use
the internet to find out about yoga for seniors and how to adapt it to a
variety of situations.

Also, there are many types of meditation and visualization that have
become popular over the last 50 years. My personal recommendation,
based on over 40 years of experience, is to look into Transcendental
Meditation or "TM" (introduced to the Western world by Maharishi
Mahesh Yogi and famously practiced by the Beatles, and more recently
Jerry Seinfeld and Oprah Winfrey, among countless other celebrities).
The American Heart Association recently endorsed TM as a very effective modality in the reduction of hypertension, and recommended this
technique for those who may have concerns about high blood pressure.
Recall with over 100 million Americans who display pre-diabetes or
diabetes, hypertension may be a significant factor in how well (or not)
we age. For more information on TM, go to *www.TM.org.*

**8: A Few Supplemental Spices and Fruits.** Think of this suggestion as a compliment to diet and nutrition. A number of things I will
recommend here are great substitutes for salt and sugar, and tend to
make the food that is more "life-supporting" tastier, as well. The first is
turmeric, which is known for its anti-inflammatory qualities. Cinnamon

has been hailed as a substance that helps to prevent the formation of those neurofibrillary tangles we discussed previously. And believe it or not, berries (both strawberries and blueberries) seem to help inhibit the buildup of amyloid plaque, which is one of the key hallmarks of Alzheimer's disease. (Not to mention they taste good, too.) We'll discuss more about supportive supplements in our upcoming chapter on resources.

**9: Stay informed.** The world of aging and longevity is changing daily. Illuminating resources are cropping up all over—in bookstores, on the internet and on many TV shows—regarding how we age, how to stay young, how to support our parents and how to keep up with the process of transformation. Here are some places I suggest you check out:

- *ChangingAging.com*: Dr. Bill Thomas has a very different view of how to transition into elderhood, and how our aging can look and feel different, if we make different choices than our predecessors.
- State and federal "departments of aging," which are full of statistics about how many dimensions of life are changing as our population ages.
- *Ageinplace.org* is an advocate for better quality aging services, as well as the time honored AARP, which is extremely well organized and is one of the oldest organizations of its type.
- Do a "Google-search" on the internet by typing in the "Search" bar: changing aging. There, you'll find any number of resources on the subject.
- Lastly, take a look at our newly organized BodyEnergyinstitute.org website, which is designed to be a clearinghouse for all of the subjects discussed above.

**10: Let your voice be heard.** A fair question, in response to all of the points mentioned above, is: "All of this sounds great, but how do we pay for it?" This leads us to consider how and in what way we can best enact social and cultural change. Recently, the Cancer Treatment Centers of America have included meditation and massage as legitimate parts of the treatment protocol for cancer recovery, and so they are now covered by insurance. While we, as a society, are in the beginning stages of looking at alternatives for the treatment of Alzheimer's and dementia, we *can* learn from how the process of change has occurred in the past. The example provided by the Cancer Treatment Centers of America offers us a window through which we can see other similar options—like CST, dietary and nutritional guidance, etc.—being embraced as viable, safe and effective treatment protocols for use in addressing Alzheimer's and dementia. Ultimately, we can envision these being paid for by insurance or governmental health agencies.

Obviously, a significant portion of this process of change will always be economically driven. But if you are moved to do so, I urge you to send an email or letter to your insurance provider, asking them to include in their coverage the alternative techniques we've presented here—such as craniosacral therapy—as preventative measures in the fight against Alzheimer's and dementia. It very may well end up being one of the best investments of a few minutes of your time, especially if you have a loved one who has Alzheimer's or dementia.

For a moment, consider what our country would be like if Medicare and Medicaid *were* to include these alternative therapies in their list of approved treatment modalities. My sense is that a *vast* amount of money and resources would be saved by every US taxpayer. And, it's NOT impossible to see it happening in this generation! In this day and age, with the internet and social media exponentially connecting us as a worldwide community, I believe cultural change can occur at a more rapid pace than any of us can possibly imagine!

In this chapter, we have discussed the dynamics and challenges in and around prevention, which is a subject in and of itself. In the next chapters, we will look at how we can assist those in whom the process of aging has accelerated, by exploring the concepts of *reversal and regeneration.*

Chapter **11**

# How We Heal: A Pound of Cure

After last chapter's discussion of prevention, now we turn to the topic of reversal and repair of Alzheimer's disease and dementia. Unfortunately, even though most of us know in theory that it's better to take care of ourselves and be healthy, oftentimes we have not been provided with the knowledge and/or support to live life in a healthy manner. As we age into our later years, the result of this *can* become what we call "pathological" aging (defined as "the aging of the brain being premature to the aging of the body" and is inclusive of symptoms associated with onset of Alzheimer's and dementia). When we pass the threshold from normal to pathological aging, a different conversation is in order. Spoiler Alert: reversal of the pathological aging process *is* possible, but time and commitment are essential to such a reversal. At this point, both the patient and the health care practitioner also typically make a transition from preventative to acute care medicine, from both the traditional and alternative points of view.

Let's take a look at some of the factors that contribute to pathological aging:

1. Stress: both in its general form and more localized forms
2. Toxicity: within the individual and the environment
3. Inflammation: contributes to a variety of symptoms in both the mind and body

4.  Diet: intertwined with all of the above

5.  Belief Systems: can reinforce all of the above and add to emotional stress (see #1 above)

Delving deeper, we can examine why healing from the effects of pathological aging takes time *and* may require a pound of cure, referring to Dr. Ornish's modern proverb, "An ounce of prevention is worth a pound of cure.*" (*: Basically, this means if a person is regularly and holistically caring for themselves, they will recover from a health issue that comes up easier than someone who has neglected their health and has more hurdles to jump over.) The "pound of cure" I will explain below refers to the 'why and how' it takes time to intelligently apply craniosacral therapy *and* other therapies to reverse the effect of years of neglect and intentional or unintentional abuse to the body.

Now, a fair question to ask is, "If this modern-day proverb is so obvious, why don't people take better care of themselves (the 'ounce of prevention') to avoid long-term illness?" Well, the answer may lie in how the general population is informed about what creates health *and* what does not create health. As an example, we can consider the impact of diabetes in the US (which I've previously mentioned). If there are almost 100 million people in the US who are diabetic or pre-diabetic (which in many cases can lead to heart disease and worse), one would think a rational, "health-minded" person would avoid behaviors that would create these conditions. However, so often there is something missing in a person's 'health awareness'—in this case, the necessary information (or education) showing the connection between diet, inflammation and diabetes. In fact, it seems all too common to find the difference between someone remaining healthy or developing a health issue is some important piece (or pieces) of information *that the general public is simply not aware of.*

How about another example of the prevalence of misguided information about "healthy self-care"? Many people think, *If I exercise more, that will help regulate my weight.* No doubt this is *generally* true...but as Dr. William Davis points out in his book, *Wheat Belly,* in this day and age people can run a marathon and still carry 10–20 pounds more average weight than their parents did. Perhaps here, there is another missing link, like the fact that some foods ("normal" bread, in particular, and its relationship with wheat) can create more and more inflammation in the body and make it harder to lose weight (regardless of one's exercise regimen). Perpetuating this cycle effectively contributes to pre-diabetes, or 'diabesity.' Unfortunately, it might be hard to change behavior *if* the foods we eat make us, at least temporarily, feel better. Typically, we continue (I know because I have been one of those) to maintain a diet until it eventually leads to problems, especially in old age. And then, if we want to change our living style, it can take a real commitment and change of attitude. Hence, a 'pound of cure.' But you may ask, are we ever too old to heal? (The answer, by the way, is: "No, we are *never* too old to heal.")

Most of us know intuitively that aches, pains and other bodily dysfunctions typically do not just happen overnight. Indeed, my research on Alzheimer's and dementia revealed decades of prior disease processes, such as diabetes, obesity, arthritis, cardiovascular problems and other maladies that we can connect to the inflammatory process. Whether these be from diet, trauma or a variety of other factors, the longer that stress erodes and settles in our body, the longer it make may take to leave. However, my assertion is that, just like with cardiac and diabetic dysfunction, it is possible to reverse the effects of Alzheimer's and dementia, which stand at the apex of the dysfunctional iceberg.

Physiologically speaking, here are some of the basic elements of the mechanism of pathological aging:

1. Over the course of time (decades), a person's body accumulates toxins. This is a more mechanical way of describing how we store stress.

2. These toxins, in time, cause localized and/or general inflammation in the body.

3. If this inflammation persists, it may affect the immune system and its ability to defend itself. An example of this continued inflammatory response and immune system interaction is autoimmune dysfunction, such as rheumatoid arthritis, what some cardiologists such as Dr. Mark Houston term an "auto-immune disease" and what I have described in the advanced stages of Alzheimer's. Also, my most recent treatment experience has led me to believe that multiple sclerosis (MS) can

certainly reflect an inflammatory process in the body, albeit affecting different structures in the body than Alzheimer's and dementia. In the case of MS specifically, the protective nerve coating, called myelin, within the central nervous system is affected. Coupled to this is the observation that, in many of these patients, diet may play a role in just how severely the symptoms display themselves. Eventually, the contribution of inflammatory producing elements in the diet may accelerate an autoimmune response within the immune system and the body begins to attack itself. The same observation could be made about rheumatoid arthritis, where inflammatory diet factors may help contribute to the immune system's overreaction and an autoimmune response is generated.

4.  Another consequence of continued inflammation in the body is tissue damage. This also relates to the cross linkage and random damage theories I referred to earlier (I discussed cross linkage in Chapter 10, along with the theories of normal aging). This continued inflammation, which can result in tissue damage, may be because of insufficient blood supply or a combination of other factors, including the inflammatory influences of certain types of food. Damaged tissues may be localized or general. They can be in an organ, such as the liver, spleen, pancreas, kidneys, eyes, heart, stomach or the GI tract. Indeed, depending on how widespread the damage, the whole body can become involved, even affecting the cellular mitochondria and our ability to use energy in an effective way.

5.  An additional consequence and reflection of tissue damage (which can, again, be caused by continued inflammation) is calcification. We are most familiar with this in relation to the cardiovascular system, as it was commonly called "hardening of the arteries" in times past. And yet this calcification occurs not just in the arteries, but in the veins and the entire network of the vascular system, which supplies life-giving blood to our brain and body.  The calcification process begins with cholesterol, which shows up in response to the need for protecting the arteries and veins from inflammation. The veins and arteries

become coated with more and more cholesterol, which results in a continuing loss of flexibility in the vascular transport system of the body. That is, over time, the veins and arteries lose their inherit ability to be supple, flexible and able to respond readily to a wide variety of situations. I recently saw an interview of former President Bill Clinton by CNN's Wolf Blitzer. Mr. Clinton shared how he had received a stint in his artery, and yet it was clogging up or closing off yet again. That motivated him to undertake "the pound of cure" program which, in this case, was the functional medicine alternatives proposed by Dr. Mark Hyman, to avoid any further complications. Former President Clinton apparently had to experience the fear of death to motivate him to change his diet and lifestyle. However, now he looks and says he feels years younger. I mention this as additional evidence that healing is possible. My wish for all and a primary reason I wrote this book is to *prevent a health crisis before the pound of cure is necessary.*

6. Finally, and intertwined with the above, nerve damage can occur as a result of pathological aging. Examples of this can range from multiple sclerosis to fibromyalgia, erectile dysfunction, diabetes and moderate and advanced stages of Alzheimer's and dementia.

On a personal note, one of the reasons I am so focused on reversal of the aging process and, indeed, understanding the steps of how we heal, is for my own well-being. After a year or more of teaching classes on longevity and doing research on diabetes, heart disease and Alzheimer's, it slowly dawned on me that perhaps all of this had some personal relevance. It brought to mind the well-known term, "Walk your talk." I must admit I took as much time as I could avoiding the subject. However, I understand the nature of avoidance, denial and resistance extremely well. Nevertheless, I was motivated by a number of factors (not the least of which was/is a beautiful young daughter who I would like to see continue to grow, flower and unfold in her extraordinary life). So, with the gentle suggestion of an associate of mine, Dr. Tim Hutton, I took the plunge and began exploring and eventually embraced functional medicine as part of my own health regimen.

The result for me has been encouraging, perhaps even astonishing. As I mentioned at the beginning of this book, in 4 months I lost 24 pounds and dramatically reduced my blood panels, including my A1c levels and other indicators of cardiovascular health. I've learned how to cook and make diet choices that work, even while traveling, from Canada to Moscow and beyond. I can say I had taken myself right to the border of pathological aging without going over the edge. But that was close enough for me. I am not yet complete in my own healing process, but I am well on the way. A friend of mine from West Virginia once said to me, "My daddy would say you've been living high on the hog, Michael." High on the hog, indeed.

Yes, I have my own personal experience of what it takes to reverse years of abuse, being a Baby Boomer and living through the sixties. I also realize that my own belief systems have been challenged, and I would not want anyone to do what I myself have not been willing to do. As a result of this experience, I am gaining hope and a sense of possibility. I can see a future of good heath, vibrant life, expansion and love. I also understand the nature of patience in allowing the history of the past to heal itself. It is in this spirit that I discuss the next section, the stages of healing. This is a model I've developed, as I've continued working in our craniosacral mini-intensive programs around the country.

### The Three Stages of Healing Alzheimer's:
### Metaphorically Extinguishing a Forest Fire in the Brain

It came to me that the best way to explain what I consider to be the three stages of the healing process for Alzheimer's is to compare it to—especially in relation to Alzheimer's and dementia—putting out a forest fire. Although not an expert in this area, growing up in southern California and traveling in Montana has given me some visual experience of what extinguishing a forest fire involves.

Let's start by recalling, we have discussed rather extensively the inflammatory nature of Alzheimer's and dementia. If any condition fits the bill for brain inflammation, Alzheimer's would be the one. Indeed, think of Alzheimer's as brain inflammation that's out of control, or soon to be out of control. Now, we all know what happens when a forest fire is unmanaged and runs its course. It will consume every available resource until it burns itself out, leaving thousands of acres destroyed in the process, the land having become empty and fallow. Alzheimer's, in its full progression, basically does the same thing. It consumes healthy brain issue and leaves behind desiccated, non-functional, non-viable tissue. Death is the ultimate result.

### Reversal of Alzheimer's and Dementia—A Bold Proposal

I call the BodyEnergy Longevity Prescription "a bold proposal," because it is exactly that.

Before laying out the proposal itself, let me speak about healing a bit more. Based on my experience with thousands of clients, I've seen how the improvement of one's state of health, that is, healing, moves in stages, in a gradual and positive way, whether it be with children with autism, older adults with traumatic brain injury, Vietnam vets with PTSD or patients with chronic headaches and migraines. Because of this, it is necessary to note that, in following through with this proposal, not everyone will necessarily see the degree of improvement they would like in the timeframe they'd hope for. Still, I can say that the vast majority have seen significant improvement and increased quality of life. It is this potential for change that drives my proposal that Alzheimer's and dementia could be reversed.

Given the rather bleak picture of what Alzheimer's looks like in its full state of progression, how do we dare approach the inflammatory issue? According to my proposal, just as in fighting a forest fire, we contain it and prevent expansion. This is the first phase, stopping the momentum. In the next phase, we actually extinguish or significantly extinguish the blaze, and one technique is to remove the fuel or dry tinder that feeds the fire. This is the second, or stabilizing and reversal phase. Thirdly, we repair the damage, as in reseeding a forest once it has been consumed or partially consumed. This is the third or repair stage. I'll now elaborate upon all of the stages, with a focus on Alzheimer's.

## Stages of Healing

**Phase 1:** *Stop the momentum and contain the blaze*
(three to six months)

Think of the slide towards pathological or accelerated aging as a blazing fire slowly beginning to smolder and burn. That is, there are outer indications of this "negative momentum," including multiple symptoms, multiple conditions or diagnoses, and perhaps even multiple medications one may try in order to hold the line for a distressed patient. The timing of the onset of this negative momentum can vary greatly with each individual. Some see a gradual decline, while for others, it's as if

### How CranioSacral Therapy Can Reverse the Aging Process

CST is an excellent way to address several key aspects by providing four main benefits:

#### 1. Increase CSF volume
* *clears heavy metals across the blood brain barrier*
* *protects the brain from inflammatory processes*
* *influence the health of the neuro-skeletal-muscular-vascular system*

#### 2. Increase fluid flow
* *relaxes connective tissue*
* *positively influences vision and related structures*
* *strengthens connective tissue fluid flow and the character of the skin*
* *increases oxygen intake and therefore positively impacts respiratory function and overall energy*
* *supports increased muscle elasticity*
* *lowers blood pressure*
* *increases nutrient absorption*
* *improves overall aerobic metabolism to the brain and body for repair and maintenance*
* *helps promote detoxification*

#### 3. Affects immune and endocrine system function
* *improves the ratio of bone production and reabsorption*
* *improves and promotes red blood cell health and platelet production factors*
* *promotes protein synthesis*
* *enhances endocrine and pituitary function*
* *promotes more balanced liver and gall bladder function*
* *promotes more balances pancreatic and insulin function*

#### 4. Creates neurological balance
* *addresses deep structures within the central nervous system*
* *stabilizes sleep patterns*
* *promotes a healthier cardiac rhythm*
* *improves balance and vestibular control*

multiple symptoms and conditions appear out of nowhere. This is in all probability an indication of how much inherent resource, or biological age, that patient has at any one time. Unfortunately, by the time brain inflammation is clearly evident, the fire is well underway, which makes the "pound of cure" approach somewhat justified.

Using mild to moderate Alzheimer's as an example, our proposed approach for stopping its momentum is to initially offer an intervention that is fast, easily applied and non-traumatizing to the patient. Applying a craniosacral StillPoint once a day, for five to ten minutes, will typically be enough to show some initial change after about three weeks. Given the positive effects of this protocol are cumulative, it's highly likely continued application will show even greater progress.

At this stage, this first step will be enough to get our foot in the door. Remember, these are patients who have, knowingly or unknowingly, carried decades of inflammation in their bodies. Even quelling their agitation or bringing some moments of silence is significant to the quality of their lives (not to mention their caregiver's, as well). Just as important is the quality or change in their communication and behavior, something which their family typically can see and about which they begin to feel hopeful. In this stage of the healing process, several levels of the patient's life are being simultaneously affected.

On the level of the physiology, the body is beginning to experience the first stages of reduced inflammation. Depending on the stage and progression of the disease's momentum, it may have gained considerable headway. Nevertheless, with consistency of treatment, the body has an opportunity to, at the very least, take a pause and feel the effects of inner rest without immune system chaos and inflammation. Additionally, during the craniosacral StillPoint therapy, the accumulated toxicity from years of wear and tear, not to mention any side effects of multiple medications, has an opportunity to be released and safely exit the body. Just as the firefighters douse a forest fire with massive amounts of water, the increased flow of cerebrospinal fluid during a CST session literally bathes the brain in more fluid, sending nourishing CSF to all parts of the central nervous system. Additionally, the tendency of the brain to dry out, which is highly accelerated in dementia and advanced dementia patients, begins to change the brain's character. Brain and membrane tissue, however, have the ability to become

more viable, in the same way we discussed reversing the effects of calcification with cardiovascular disease.

With continued CST sessions for the Alzheimer's patient, his or her
family members and care-givers can expect to enjoy improved psychol-
ogies, as they begin observing positive changes and differences in the
patient's communication and/or behavior. This is certainly an important element in the healing process, because the family and community
then have an opportunity to entertain changing their own belief systems, based upon seeing something positive happen, and not just a
continual downward momentum. After all, it's likely no one has ever
shared with them the notion, "Positive change is possible," especially in
a condition of this severity. Just seeing "a break in the clouds" can be an
important step for everyone involved.

I know in my own experience working with children diagnosed
with autism, a parent is frequently told no change is possible, leaving
that parent with a feeling of hopelessness. So, when in that context,
after a number of craniosacral treatments, one hears the first word
ever spoken by the child and sees the tears in the parent's eyes, it's evident that change is *indeed* possible.

On yet another level, administrative awareness has an opportunity
to change. When the manager of a facility begins to notice there are less
patient complaints, that the staff find it easier to work with residents,
and that friends and relatives visit more often and enjoy their visits
more, they can begin to see how this translates into overall improvement in quality of life. It then becomes easier to extrapolate how this
could have a positive multiplying effect across the entire facility (even
the economic "bottom line" would likely improve, due to decreased
staff stress and corresponding stress-related costs).

On an emotional level, there is an additional subtle, but significant
result of this proposed therapeutic program. The years of emotion a
patient with Alzheimer's has experienced that are often intertwined
with the toxicity of the body can be silently acknowledged. One of
the things I observed in our initial study was the increased awareness of the residents we were treating, when relaxation and listening
became available, even after just ten minutes of the administration of
a StillPoint. Physiologically, we say this lowers sympathetic tone and,
therefore, one of the observed benefits is a diminishing of agitation. In

addition to this physical change, the emotions locked deep inside an Alzheimer's patient may finally find a way to exit the body in a safe and noninvasive way. As this process continues day after day, more of the patient's true, detoxified emotions can naturally be expressed. I fully realize the acknowledgment of emotions may not always be welcomed or understood. However, in this context, the results of the healing process can be seen as being, overall, worthy of the possible challenges along the way.

Additional benefits of this stage include gaining confidence that there are no unwanted side effects, and that, given individual resources, an easy simple intervention can produce positive change without any unwanted consequences. Starting and proceeding slowly, with the acknowledgement that the patient typically has a more sensitive and fragile physiology, sets the foundation for the next step.

**Phase 2:** *Stabilization and Reversal—Extinguish the blaze*
(six to twelve months)

Quite honestly, I would be thrilled just to see the first phase of this proposal put into practice on a significant level. By "significant" I mean, if just 2–3% of all 17,000 nursing homes in the US adopted even Phase One of this proposal, "Stop the Momentum," we would reach a significant tipping point in the treatment and approach to Alzheimer's and dementia. However, I want to outline a full program, in the hope that a vision of possibility can encourage many of us to move ahead, especially those of us who would like to substantially improve the quality of life for our senior population. It should be noted, some of the following suggestions for Phases 2 and 3 are simple, but revolutionary. In the current senior care system, some or all of this might be charted or billed under what we call "private pay."

**How do we put out the blaze of brain inflammation?**
Here are the steps:

1. *Administration of the StillPoint*
We continue what we have begun in Phase 1, regular administration of the StillPoint. When and if possible, we add to the frequency of CST treatment, increasing to two or three times a day. This is where friends,

family and volunteers can also be of assistance. In our firefighting analogy, it would be equivalent to enlisting more firefighters and calling for
aerial support to come in to assist in the quelling of the blaze. Bringing
in additional help also has the effect of increasing the momentum of the
healing process and, in all probability, shortening the timeline to see
results, i.e., the patient's gradual recovery of his or her brain and body.
Literally, there is more fluid on a CSF and interstitial level to quell the
inflammation. To be fair, I am stretching the analogy here a bit. It's not as
if we are hosing down inflammatory agents of cytokines in the brain and
body, although I have had patients describe it in precisely that way. However, the point is this: the effect of increased fluid flow of CSF produces a
similar effect, washing the brain of inflammatory agents and toxins that
cause—as Alzheimer's progresses—those amyloid precursor proteins
(APP's) to miscode and create the beta and gamma amyloid plaques,
which ultimately destroy brain tissue. Our goal here is to interrupt the
process, slow the progression and ultimately stop it altogether.

2.  *Additional CST support*

Our CST practitioners, including those trained in the initial two-day
class or CSLAD, have learned specific therapeutic techniques, including
the StillPoint, and other approaches that can be done over a period of 30
minutes with each patient. They can easily hone in on problem areas in
the brain and body, and eliminate those "hot pockets" where inflammatory agents have clustered and provide the ground to spread to other
areas. Oftentimes, it seems the pre-frontal lobe is where inflammation
is initially found, at least this is so with Alzheimer's. This is, unfortunately, also one of the more vulnerable parts of the brain, the one that
is the latest to develop and is instrumental in creating judgment and
planning for the future. It is no wonder, then, that dementia patients
live more in the past and do not have ready access to the future. This
is a reflection of what osteopaths refer to as "structure and function,"
and reflects how the different parts of brain physiology support specific behaviors. Our goal here is to zero in on the most vulnerable areas
and support recovery in an easy, comfortable way.

3.  *Diet and nutrition*

Here we enter into a sensitive area, but there is simply no way
around it. In stopping a forest fire, one way to stop the blaze is to

remove the fuel in the path of the fire, especially if that fuel is dry tinder ready to explode. If the fuel that is feeding the fire can be removed, there is a greater probability the fire will die out by itself. Less fuel, less fire. The hard truth is that many foods we eat are inflammatory in nature and have been creating inflammation and toxicity for decades in our senior population. That's why leaders in the health field, such as Drs. Dean Ornish, Mark Hyman, Andrew Weil and others are starting to call Alzheimer's "type 3 diabetes." We have already spent a good deal of time discussing this, but I'll just review some of the main concepts. Recall insulin resistance and metabolic syndrome. Over time, this inflammation can not only flood the body—hardening the arteries and causing autoimmune diseases and diabetes—but ultimately, in at least some cases, it overflows into the brain. Many foods seem suspect in their ability to trigger an inflammatory response, including excesses of sugar, as well as wheat in many forms. This is currently the subject of a great deal of research, which I've discussed in Chapter 8.

Now, let's take a step back. I realize food choices are a personal matter, with every individual basing his or her decisions about what to eat on a wide variety of factors. I also understand the concept of "comfort food." After all, I've spent most of my life allowing food to soothe and anesthetize me, and be even a reward for achievement or a substitute for love. When we, as adults, even *suggest* that soda past a certain size be banned in New York City, or that school cafeterias be required to offer more healthy choices, public outcry can ensue. However, there are some chilling statistics staring us in the face, such as 100 million Americans being pre-diabetic. That's about one in three, and predicted to go as high as one in two over time. That's not just a statistic, people...*that's an epidemic!*

I also don't want to suggest that we should take away the favorite foods our parents or grandparents enjoy at home or in assisted living facilities or nursing homes. It turns out, though, that some of the most tasty, habit-forming and addictive foods are the most inflammatory. (It's almost as if someone had designed them that way.) After all, we probably feel badly enough that our loved one is in the condition they're in. Consciously or unconsciously, it is common to show love for others in the way we provide or share food. It is, and probably always will be, a way to say, "Mom (or Dad), I love you," without having to say the words.

I'd like to pose a few questions, however, "What if there could be a diet of *healthy* (God forbid, I should use this word), tasty food for the senior population, especially those in any stage of dementia and Alzheimer's? And what if they actually liked it? And, to be even more bold, what if it didn't cost significantly more for a facility to purchase and prepare such foods?" Allow yourself a few moments to reflect on this vision of possibilities—how might this change the quality of life for those living with Alzheimer's and dementia?

Well, this is exactly what the BodyEnergy Institute for Longevity and Quality of Life is currently developing, with the assistance of expert health care professionals in this field. Since education is key in this area, we are partnering with those trained in holistic nutrition to develop cost-effective, compelling (tasty) meals, and creating a food preparation program for those who are working in institutional settings. As part of this process and as a clearinghouse for more information, BodyEnergy-institute.org (*www.BodyEnergyinstitute.org*) has been created to update anyone interested in the latest information on diet, therapist availability, research and the newest developments in our Longevity program.

Certainly, adopting this proposed non-inflammatory diet will require educating family members and caregivers, as well as nursing home and assisted living facility administrators, all of whom may struggle with the same issues surrounding food. Remember, the statistics for those who are pre-diabetic are one in three.

Let me provide one example of how this could work. The CEO of Safeway (a North American grocery store), Steve Burd, started to look at corporate healthcare costs and saw they were topping over $1 billion a year. He then began to look at ways these costs could be contained or at least prevented from going any higher. Safeway started to introduce healthier food choices in their cafeterias, and gave "health credits" to their employees for weight loss, lowering of blood pressure, decreased cholesterol, etc. In essence, he incentivized healthy and positive well-being behavior. The result? To date, Safeway has saved over $100 million annually in health care costs. To quote Mr. Burd, "Making money and doing something good are not mutually exclusive."

What are some of the physiological impacts of a non-inflammatory diet? For one, weight loss. As pro-inflammatory foods are removed from the diet, the swelling in the tissue literally goes down. Metaphorically speaking, the dry tinder fueling the forest fire begins to be removed. Recall that adipose (fat cells) create their own inflammation in the form of pro-inflammatory adipocykines or adipokines. When one's diet is stripped of these inflammatory elements and the body begins to adapt to a different type of fat-burning mechanism, the adipose tissue naturally starts to be consumed. I know this from personal experience. With the proper nutritional and supplement support, the body mass index or BMI also begins to shift. And when one adds proper exercise to the mix, there is the possibility of greater muscle mass, which will also promote a healthier metabolism and more efficient fat-burning.

An additional benefit of a healthier, non-inflammatory diet is less cardiac congestion and excess fluid around vital cardiovascular structures—what we often see in congestive heart failure. In seniors with increased health challenges, cardiac congestion is often one of the final aspects of pathological aging that reinforces their immobility and lessens their energy.

At this point, I'd like to address one other factor. We have all observed seniors who seem sedentary and overweight. On the other hand, we can easily find ourselves associating "aging" with people looking thin and frail—especially those with medical complications. I had a lesson in this when volunteering at Robin Lim's (CNN's 2011 "Hero of the Year") free clinic in Ubud, on the island of Bali in Indonesia. Besides doing great work promoting healthy pregnancies in the region, Ms. Lim also invites people in need to her clinic, many of them family members and grandparents of the pregnant mother. I noticed that many of the thin men and women coming for assistance had the symptoms of congestive heart failure and pronounced edema (swelling) in the chest, legs and other extremities. I was puzzled at first, until Robin explained this was not uncommon in many regions of Indonesia. Rice has long been a staple of this population. However, a few decades ago, international health authorities introduced a strain of rice that was eventually found to produce the swelling and inflammation I have been discussing.

The point of this story is to illustrate that, even in the US, many outwardly thin people are actually starving for proper nutrition. Dr. Mark Hyman, in his book, *The Blood Sugar Solution* points out that any number of thin people can be pre-diabetic, as well. This also transfers to our senior population. Dr. Bill Thomas, the founder of innovative senior care facilities named Eden Alternatives and the more recent Green House Projects, made the same point about seniors in an interview I conducted with him in 2013. Dr. Thomas said, "Sudden weight loss is an indicator of problems for seniors and always poses a danger to senior residents. Proper nutrition and a healthy diet, including when and how a senior eats, can make a difference in the overall well-being of an elderly patient."

There are yet more benefits to being on an anti-inflammatory diet, especially with the population challenged with dementia and Alzheimer's. Recall I also discussed the progression of the stages of inflammation that leads to moderate to severe Alzheimer's. I mentioned the acute phase response as an adaptation to chronic inflammation, such that the body and brain can exhibit an anaerobic response, social withdrawal, and a change in endocrine function. As inflammation is reduced, these symptoms also have an opportunity to be reduced, the result being even greater metabolic balance (which is key in regulating blood sugars), as well as an improved ability to interact with the outside world. Also, proteins and peptides that regulate digestion, inflammation and, ultimately, energy to the brain, begin to fall into more appropriate homeostatic balance. A downshifting in all of the above lessens cardiovascular and diabetes risk factors, not to mention giving the brain "space and time" as it heals. In essence, the blaze starts to be extinguished.

4.  *Supplements*

There is much I can say about this, and indeed, I will go into more detail in the chapter on resources. The key idea, especially in relation to the senior population, is that there are natural vitamins and minerals that can help support the body in its healing process, as inflammation decreases. These supplements, which obviously must be selected somewhat specifically for each person, can help correct imbalances in the mind-body system, even if they have existed for many years. As an added benefit, supplements may also support healthy psychological behavior, or simply put, reduce depression that at least in some patents, may have been mistaken for dementia.

5.  *Exercise*

I'm not suggesting that an eighty- or ninety-year-old go out and try to run a four-minute mile, although there are seniors who are in remarkable physical shape. However, the sedentary lifestyle that we see all too often in senior care has the potential of being shifted. As an example, while teaching in the beautiful and charming city of Halifax, Nova Scotia, Canada, I discovered tai chi for seniors. It is a practice of gentle, intentional focus and stretching that strengthens the cardio-vascular system and promotes increasing flexibility in the body. It was wonderful to witness a group of seniors, from ages 70–90, gracefully and easily moving their bodies in a harmonious and wise way. There is a practitioner in that area who has developed a tai chi practice that helps reduce the symptoms of arthritis, as well.

Another example of exercise for seniors with Alzheimer's is Pilates. In the 1920's and 30's, the German-born Joseph Pilates developed a revolutionary physical fitness system that can be used even while lying in a hospital bed. By sharing this system with bedridden patients during WWI, Pilates taught them how to strengthen themselves and assist in their own healing process toward full physical recovery. It should be noted Pilates believed that mental and physical health are interrelated.

Exercise of the type I am suggesting can even be modified for patients who are wheelchair-bound, and some programs have been developed taking this into consideration. One such resource can be found at _http://www.helpguide.org/life/workouts_exercise_overweight_ _disabled.htm_. One of the resources I'll mention in the next chapter suggests that half an hour a day of walking or exercise in itself may be an excellent measure to prevent the onset of Alzheimer's. In conjunction with an anti-inflammatory diet, gentle exercise modified as appropriate to a senior population can reinforce the positive momentum, while the blaze of inflammatory fires are quelled. Physiologically, there is simply less opportunity for pro-inflammatory pockets to hide and fester in the body, and therefore even less opportunity for the diminishing "dry tinder" in the brain and body to ignite. At present, the BodyEnergy Institute is working with healthcare professionals to develop exercise programs and similar resources specifically tailored for at-home use and live-in facility applications.

6.  *Attending physician support*

Indeed, the reduction of inflammation caused by changes in diet and administration of CST may create a new and important role for the doctor looking after the medication of each patient. Instead of reviewing an Alzheimer's patient's medications on a monthly or bimonthly basis, while presiding over a gradual and inevitable decline of mental and physical health, the attending doctor may now be focused on *finding* signs of positive change and improvement. This is vital, I believe, as an alternative to the prevailing model, in which a doctor would simply never expect or even look for a patient's improvement.

The number of physicians practicing gerontological medicine—the study of and specialization in the aging population—is relatively small in the US. However, it is projected that 36,000 new geriatricians will be needed by 2030, which to many seems to be an unrealistic expectation. In point of fact, 80% of pediatric patients see pediatricians, while 80% of geriatric patents see primary care doctors or internists, according to Dr. Gregg Warshaw of the University of Cincinnati, author of a report on the demographics of this situation. This statistic points out the need to recognize that monitoring and improvement of seniors' health and quality of life is a specialty in and of itself. In a very real sense, a team approach utilizing a broader base of healthcare professionals is needed, as suggested by further reports and studies. Our partners in the medical profession need to recognize that the differences in an aging population will help support and redefine what aging is and what opportunities for improved well-being and quality of life are available.

The area of senior healthcare is still an emerging field and a doctor who is thrust into this unfamiliar area might not readily have all the answers. This puts the onus on *us,* actually, to educate ourselves for the best care of our loved one. I've had friends who, knowing full well the history of their parents, made positive recommendations about treatment of mom and dad to the attending physician...with good results! (Parents who consult with a pediatrician about their children are familiar with this sort of dynamic and interaction.) As the field of senior healthcare develops, it gives us an opportunity to create a new dynamic and conversation between healthcare providers, the patient, and the caregiver and family. Honest, open-minded communication between all these parties may create an altogether new direction in treatment and quality of life for our seniors.

Regarding my experience utilizing craniosacral therapy in the pediatric population, I've seen that our own specialization in this area has emerged and refined itself over the last 20 years. And so it is with our "Longevity" program, as well. I will elaborate on this in greater detail when I make further suggestions about senior care reform.

7.   *Blood work and other physiological measures*

I am taking a page here from functional medicine. The use of bloodwork and other physiological measures presents an exciting opportunity to verify and validate the effects of my proposed suggestions outlined above. Functional medicine looks at the interrelationship of all body systems, not just a singular specialized approach. One way for a physician to monitor progress is to conduct an extensive series of blood panel tests that monitor and reveal the extent of insulin resistance, blood sugars and a variety of other factors. In this way, a doctor can objectively evaluate the impact of a non-inflammatory diet on the body over time, whether it be over the course of weeks, months or years. (The same could be done for exercise or any of the other proposed elements of the BodyEnergy Longevity Prescription for Alzheimer's.)

Because the underlying assumption of the current medical model has been that decline over a gradual period of time is the rule of thumb for people with Alzheimer's, there has not been a lot of data collected to indicate what recovery or improvement looks like. However, a good many of these measures are objective, experimentally derived and have been established as guidelines for the younger general population. For example, a functional medicine doctor may order traditional and some non-traditional blood tests that include the evaluation of LDL, triglycerides, blood sugar levels and insulin resistance, as well as taking the traditional blood pressure level. With these measures, they are then able to assess the effects of dietary changes and the addition of specific supplements. We believe this same assessment technique can be applied to seniors, as well, including the Alzheimer's population. With the advent and adoption of the BodyEnergy Longevity Prescription, there is an opportunity to establish new measures and standards for this population. We could, in all practicality, modify the frequency and degree of these measurements to our population. Based on our example above, doctors skilled in the observation of their senior populations could discover what other blood work reflects a positive change. This is an in-process proposal, and involves the partnership of the senior care medical community in developing these new protocols. In my mind, the question is, "What if we could validate that, over time, specific changes in diet and exercise, along with regular sessions of craniosacral therapy, to name just a few of our suggestions, would result in significant improvements in Alzheimer's patients' physiology?" Following that line of thinking, a number of other questions arise: "Would the effects of this protocol eventually make a difference in the way, amount or kind of Alzheimer's medication is administered? Would this sort of evaluation of effects take this proposed therapeutic program out of the realm of conjecture and into verifiable reality? Could a research study of the proposed BodyEnergy Longevity Prescription be conducted and the results evaluated, such that it might even be discovered that recovery from Alzheimer's and reversal of damage to nerves and tissue is possible?

My point is, using this proposed 'Stage 2' program allows us to monitor, over time, how hot the fires of inflammation are burning and more objectively monitor progress on an individual level.

8.    *Case history and reporting*

Finally, there is one more way to help monitor our progress in extinguishing the blaze of inflammation. The BodyEnergy Institute is working with physical therapists, occupational therapists and speech therapists to develop a model case history report, as we continue treating and supporting Alzheimer's and dementia patients. These case histories are certainly not as formal as a full-blown scientific study, but they do add valuable insight into how individuals and groups respond to all the suggestions discussed above. By chronicling, evaluating and publishing for review a thorough and well-documented collection of case histories, we can all learn together, and share this experience and information to increase the pace of our progress. A case history template has been developed and is available to healthcare practitioners for use in their particular facility or practice. It can be downloaded by going to: *http://BodyEnergy.net/case-history-template*.

Chapter **12**

# Phase 3: Regeneration—Reseeding the forest and healing the brain

In the last two chapters we've discussed the concepts of "prevention" and "reversal," as a way of understanding two of the three steps I see comprising a potential healing process for Alzheimer's and dementia. In this chapter, we'll look more deeply into what I call the final phase of this process, *regeneration.* Given the many years I've used craniosacral therapy in my practice and as an instructor at the Upledger Institute, I've come to observe that even reversal of longstanding damage to the brain and other structures is possible. I'll be providing some examples of how both I and others have achieved this and how it can become part of the third phase of our proposed treatment program, the BodyEnergy Longevity Prescription.

## 1.  Continued and enhanced treatment with CST

This third stage, regeneration of the brain and central nervous system, will likely be considered the most controversial of the three steps of what I'm proposing is a healing process for Alzheimer's and dementia. After all, many will ask, "Is it really possible to reverse, restore, and heal the effects of decades of damage to the body and brain?" Fortunately, there *is* evidence suggesting this is possible.

For the first example, I'll turn again to Dr. Dean Ornish, who has been a pioneer in the area of cardiovascular health. Over 25 years ago,

Dr. Ornish published a paper in the *New England Journal of Medicine* that documented the reversal of cardiovascular damage to the body. Yes, he met with more than a little skepticism, if not outright alarm and opposition from his fellow cardiologists. Nevertheless, his research continued to confirm his findings and today the notion that reversal and repair of cardiovascular damage is widely accepted. I actually recall a testimonial from one of Dr. Ornish's patients who, 25 years ago, was given one year to live. According to his testimonial, which was featured in the 2012 documentary film, *Escape Fire: The Fight to Save American Healthcare,* the man is still alive and well. Along with ushering in the concept of cardiovascular damage being repaired and reversed, Dr. Ornish went on to champion the cause of prevention, which, as we have seen, certainly went against the grain of the prevailing medical paradigm. It took 16 years, but Dr. Ornish's heart healthy diet program is now covered by Medicare. As Dr. Ornish says, "When a modality or treatment is covered by insurance or the medical community, it signals a sea of change in the way we look at and accept what is possible."

I'd like to share another relevant observation from Dr. Ornish, which he made during an interview with the *Huffington Post*:

> "I thought that when we published our findings in the leading medical journals that this would change medical practice. In retrospect, that was a little naïve. Good science is important, but not sufficient to change medical practice. Despite the talk about evidence-based medicine, we really live in an era of what I call 'reimbursement-based medicine,' meaning, it's all about the Benjamins. I realized that it wasn't enough to have good science. We also needed to change reimbursement. We doctors do what we get paid to do and we get trained to do what we get paid to do. Therefore, if we could change reimbursement, then we would improve both medical practice and medical education."

Now let's examine the connection between reversal of cardiovascular damage and Alzheimer's and dementia. We've previously talked about the connection between diabetes and cardiovascular disease. In the context of inflammation in the body, we have seen how this "out of control" mechanism overflows into the brain, often causing the symptoms of Alzheimer's and dementia. If we are able to put out the blaze or inflammation in the body, and then *simultaneously* create a positive effect in the brain, we could ask, "Are the same mechanisms that reverse the damage in the heart also at work in the brain?" According to Dr. Dean Ornish, Dr. David Perlmutter and others, the answer is *yes.*

As might be expected, the very same recommendations and resources I've previously discussed in Phases 1 and 2 contribute positively to the healing and reversal of Alzheimer's in Phase 3. Increased flow of cerebrospinal fluid not only irrigates the brain, but in this stage, actually helps to rebuild and reconstruct brain tissue. This has been demonstrated in a new and exciting area of brain research, which has to do with focusing on the role of glial (meaning glue) cells, the "stuffing" (as I like to call it) that surrounds, supports and envelops a great many of the axons and synapses of the brain. What is being discovered is that glial cells are actually so much more than glue. Within the realm of CSF, we actually can follow the pathways of these glial cells and their cousins, the astrocytes and oligodendrocytes, much like a drop of water might descend down a strand of a spider web. When this life-nourishing CSF, full of neurotransmitters, reaches its destination, it helps to replace and reconstruct damaged nerve tissue. Admittedly, repair of nerve tissue can take time, but its occurrence *has* recently been discussed in an article by Kendra Cherry, "Adult Neurogenesis: Can We Grow New Brain Cells?"

I would also like to include one more exciting addition to the point about glial cells, astrocytes and oligodenrocytes mentioned above. Earlier (in Chapter 4), when discussing Dr. Upledger and his Pressurestat model, I referred to recent research on the role of glymphatics, which suggested there is a secondary mechanism for the production and reabsorption of cerebrospinal fluid. This mechanism is called glymphatics (a term made from combining glia and lymphatic) and essentially describes a newly discovered system in the brain, akin to the lymphatic system in the body. The existence of this system explains how the brain is so efficient in clearing out unwanted waste products and toxins. Also, the design of the glymphatic system is of special interest to us, because it reveals the existence of a micro-network of interrelated capillary beds that transport blood (like an inner ring and an outer ring of piping) and carry CSF. The astrocytes (a specialized form of glia) draw the CSF deep within the brain via this system of glial cells. Think of this as an incredible system of micro-plumbing with connections that can virtually reach every nerve and cell within the brain.

The existence of this glymphatic system offers some new ways to look at the efficiency of CSF flow and CST treatment. The following is my theory of how these two systems complement and enhance each other:

a.  *Prevention*

If there is a mechanism that is responsible for CSF more readily improving drainage and removal of waste products from the brain, then there is the possibility that formation of plaques (made of beta amyloid) in the brain can more easily be prevented. There is a classification of neurological diseases (including amyotrophic lateral sclerosis, Alzheimer's, Parkinson's and Huntington's) that fit into a broad category called proteinopathies, a grouping which points to the existence of mis-folded or aggregated proteins. I discussed this in Chapter 2, in reference to amyloid precourser proteins that reflect this mechanism of mis-folding of the APP, resulting in formation of beta amyloid in the brain, a hallmark of Alzhiemer's disease. If techniques practiced in CST can help support increased drainage of waste products in the brain, then, as a result, formation of these plaques may be inhibited.

On the other side of the equation, increased flow and circulation of CSF occasioned by CST techniques will typically *also* assist the brain in clearing out toxicity and warding off problems associated with inflammation. In this model, both an *increase in production and increase in reabsorption* is the result.

b.  *Repair*

The same mechanism proposed above can also be seen as giving rise to the possibility of repair of brain and nervous system tissue. The glymphatic system represents a fine network of capillary beds and CSF transport, such that fresh and vital CSF, rich in neurotransmitters, can reach virtually every point in the brain. The repair of brain tissue, we can conjecture, relies on fluid transport and exchange of nutrients that lays the groundwork for repair of damaged cells and nerves on a microscopic level.

A number of other factors we have discussed can also reinforce and accelerate this process. As has been noted, nutrition *can* be medicine. In this phase, food that has helped release toxicity in Phases 1 and 2 also assists in repair. Introducing a patient-specific balance of supplements and the proper nutrition can actually help restore biochemical balance, thereby creating the optimal environment for reconstruction of brain and nervous system tissue.

## 2. Advanced dialogue with cells, body and brain

Once again, we can see the potential for reversal of Alzheimer's symptoms and restorative effects in the field of epigenetics, especially the practice of "turning off" genes that cause negative effects and "turning on" the genes that promote good health. Using an analogy, when a salamander loses a limb or a tail, it can regenerate the lost appendage. Researchers such as Dr. Robert Becker—former Director of Orthopedic Surgery at the Veterans Administration Hospital of New York and called "the father of chemically induced cellular regeneration"—have found that at certain critical times, when there is a change in the electrochemical field surrounding a salamander's severed limb, it seems to send a signal to the area telling it to begin the reconstruction process. Biologists refer to "differential gene function," which is the ability of the body, at a cellular level, to read the DNA and know whether to generate a brain cell, a bone cell, or the tissue that constitutes the tail of our previously mentioned friend, the salamander. What would it be like to actually dialogue directly with a cell, or a whole collection of cells, such as those found in the immune system, and encourage them respectfully to assist in the repair process? What would be the implications for the repair and rejuvenation process of Alzheimer's patients, if this were possible?

This is exactly what we do in Phase 3, using advanced craniosacral techniques to "dialogue" with the body and encourage healing at a cellular level. Dr. Upledger found many years ago there is an 'inner wisdom' very often available to "speak" to us within each patient. He developed this technique into what is called *"SomatoEmotional Release,"* which advanced craniosacral practitioners are trained in. Practitioners learn how to deeply "listen to the body," and find out what is significant as an issue for each person. The dialogue, or 'questions and answers' between the therapist and patient, is not necessary verbal, but given the opportunity, the body will very often share what the obstructions have been to his or her healing process. Much like a negotiator, the skilled therapist can help bring resolution to the conflict (sometimes called *disease*) within the patient's body.

Another option that has the potential for assisting in the reversal of Alzheimer's is the use of stem cells, which act like a "wild card," in the body, in that they are able to "become" any cell. Dr. Upledger found, in his research on the immune system years ago, that as an extension of the dialogue described above, one additional tool is to "speak" directly to the cells (see Chapter 4, *Dr. John Upledger Cell Talk.*) Stem cells are specialized cells within the toolkit of the immune system. In the proper circumstance and with a respectful form of "listening," stem cells can be invited to regenerate specific tissue in the body. The restorative use of stem cells is also a technique that graduates of the 4-day class, "Reversal of the Aging Process," learn how to do.

Although many may be skeptical, it's the results, I believe, that are the "proof of the pudding." Let's look at a case I'm quite familiar with. A friend of mine in Chicago who is an advanced CST practitioner, applied the stem cell technique (which I just referred to above) to an area behind his eye, and his ophthalmologist scratched her head in amazement when, after about 4 months, his tissue scans showed healthy tissue emerging, *where none had been there before.*

### 3.  Multi-hands therapy

Adding to this list of approaches in Phase 3 is what is often called "multi-hands therapy." Over the past several years, The BodyEnergy Institute has created therapeutic programs called 3-day mini-intensives, modeled after the Upledger Intensive program, during which a number of trained therapists work on one person at the same time. You can think of one of these intensive programs as an in depth spa treatment for the nervous system. Imagine for a few moments, a number of therapists all devoting their attention to the unique needs and qualities that make up the person who is resting on the table before them—this is the intensive program. I think the intensive treatment approach is one of the best things Dr. Upledger created to bring out the highest and best qualities of individually trained therapists in a group setting. It's as if the blend of individual experience and knowledge of each therapist becomes available and integrated into a cumulative and supportive "group consciousness," in order to help facilitate the healing process of the person they're attending to, no matter what the age or circumstance. The track record for our intensive program with children who have autism and cerebral palsy—conditions in and of themselves involving significant neurological challenges—has been highly encouraging. There are a large number of cases of young children regaining speech, mobility and/or the ability to communicate in a significant way. Also, the delayed development they typically experience in early years has often been significantly improved.

These very same intensive programs can also be used as a resource for seniors with Alzheimer's and dementia to aid in achieving full recovery. By Phase 3 in our proposed program, our seniors have already demonstrated the ability to regain some cognitive ability and communication skills, verified by a number of objective and subjective measures. It is at this point the opportunity to help them recover from decades of trauma is ideal. The collective, multi-hands approach we've successfully used and are herein advocating can help accelerate and clear the path for enhanced and optimum recovery, much like it has in the pediatric population.

As part of this recovery stage, let's also acknowledge the role of adult children and caregivers in this process. It would be ideal if we could share the wealth of knowledge that's been accumulated about the possible recovery from Alzheimer's with all of those who have patiently stood by and wished the best for their relatives, spouses and friends. As Dr. Leslie Cho, cardiologist at the Cleveland Clinic said, "It takes a village to make an unhealthy patient healthy." That "village" is all those who play a part in the community and support group for all our seniors. If they are open to the possibility, the same resource of multi-hands therapy is also available for them to learn, so that they might help their friend or family member peel back the layers of stress, worry and multiple challenges they have had to shoulder.

In summary, "Phase 3: Reversal—reseeding the forest and healing the brain" builds on the momentum of the practices and techniques introduced in Phases 1 and 2. We build on basic craniosacral techniques, and enhance this by increased frequency of treatment and dialogue with the immune system. In addition, we continue to build on the momentum of a healthy non-inflammatory diet, exercise and increasing mobility, all suited to recovering seniors. We also continue to biochemically monitor the changes that diet and therapy bring. Finally, we offer the resource of enhanced multi-hands therapy to accelerate recovery for our seniors and support for family and caregivers, as part of the process.

## Functioning Recovery

What I have just described is in essence the elements of what some call "functioning recovery." Here I borrow a page from therapist Tami Goldstein, who wrote a book entitled, *Coming through the Fog,* about her experiences in raising a child on the autistic spectrum. She writes about how one could have a condition called autism with sensory integration challenges, and yet can be brought to the point where they could function reasonably well, given enough patient-specific therapy and related bio-medical support for the patient *and* support from and education of family members. In Tami Goldstein's book, she makes the point that autism may be, in many cases, addressable. With the right combination of elements, her daughter is able to function reasonably well in society. This is a fairly significant departure from what many experts say is possible with children on the autistic spectrum. In a way, what she is speaking about is reversal and healing of the process of autism, at least for a specific segment of the population.

I am saying the *same* possibility of "functioning recovery" exists for those with Alzheimer's and dementia. I realize it is bold to say that the process of Alzheimer's can be halted and reversed. Certainly there may have been decades of accumulated toxicity, etc. that led to a patient's current condition. However, I propose that "functioning recovery" is a possibility—given the right combination of elements—providing a patient has sufficient support for a much improved quality of life. These elements, again, are:

| | |
|---|---|
| 1. Craniosacral therapy, on a limited and basic level | **Phase 2** |
| 2. Additional and advanced CST support | |
| 3. Diet and nutrition, another way to say a non-inflammatory diet | |

| | |
|---|---|
| 4. Supplements and biomedical support | |
| 5. Exercise and movement modified for this population | |
| 6. Attending physician support: in this case, those medical professionals who understand the role of diet and its relation to cognitive function, and who are open to monitoring change as these elements change | |
| 7. Blood work and monitoring of biochemical change, as these elements are implemented | |
| 8. Case history and reporting, to create a body of information that can be shared with other healthcare professionals as this program unfolds | |
| 9. Advanced dialogue with cells, body and brain | **Phase 3** |
| 10. Multi-hands therapy and continued advanced CST work | |

The elements above are a proposed program to approach treatment. Does one size fit all? Absolutely not. It takes, just as in the case of an autistic child, careful listening and monitoring to determine the right mix of therapies and treatments that are appropriate for each person. Additionally, given that the physiology of each senior is different and unique, differences in approach will need to be developed accordingly.

However, I believe this is a start. To propose that an advanced condition of Alzheimer's can be addressed in a positive way is bold enough, and the science and research leading up to this point warrants serious consideration.

## Chapter 13

# Drug Therapy

These next two chapters bring together resources I've mentioned throughout the book, and my elaboration upon them is mainly to support three segments of the population:

1. Seniors
2. Caregivers, for both their information and support
3. Adults of any age who would like to focus on prevention

The resources I will review not only include those associated with "alternative medicine," but also traditional medical treatments of a pharmaceutical nature, in order to give readers a perspective about how the current treatment model is used. I will also look at the progression of traditional medical treatment that may precede management of the onset of Alzheimer's and dementia. In actuality, a portion of what we will be reviewing is the drug regimen many Alzheimer's and dementia patients are and have been using—in some cases, perhaps for decades—preceding the onset of the latest phase of their disease. According to many medical authorities, these patients are sometimes classified as "medically complex," meaning they may be taking multiple medications and have multiple symptoms, the latest of which is the diagnosis of Alzheimer's and dementia.

I want to give a brief overview of some of these medications, how they work, what they target, and any long-term effects or interactions with other medications they may have. Then, I will look at alternative approaches to augment or change this traditional treatment approach. The comments below are based on my review of various research studies, journal articles and other standard medical literature. As always, consult with your physician before considering any changes in the current medications you or a relative or friend are using.

## Common Drug Treatment for Cholesterol

I'd like to begin by looking at factors that may precede the onset of Alzheimer's and dementia by decades, namely the onset of inflammation in the vascular system of the body. The most common reaction of the body to an inflammatory response is to coat the arteries and veins with cholesterol. I have discussed in some detail how various food products may accelerate this process. The solution is to lower cholesterol and related factors, choosing to target the arterial plaque buildup and not the underlying inflammatory response. The use of anti-cholesterol drugs has been a common way to lower cholesterol factors in the body. The most popular anti-cholesterol drugs used today include:

### STATIN DRUGS

Lipitor is one of the earlier statin drugs designed to lower the LDL ("bad") cholesterol and triglycerides in your blood. It can raise your HDL ("good") cholesterol, as well. Certain kinds of statin drugs (Lipitor, for example) can lower the risk of heart attack, stroke, and heart surgeries that are necessitated by cholesterol buildup in the arteries. In addition, some statin drugs can be used to decrease chest pain in patients who have heart disease or risk factors for heart disease, such as age, smoking, high blood pressure, low HDL, or family history of early heart disease.

How do statin drugs like Lipitor work? A statin is a substance that acts in the liver to block the enzyme HMG-CoA reductase. This enzyme is responsible for creating LDL cholesterol in the body. Once this cholesterol has been released from the liver, it can get trapped on the cell walls of the arteries. As the deposits grow, they trap more and more cholesterol in the artery until the artery is blocked. Lipitor reduces the amount of LDL formed, by limiting the amount of enzymes that create cholesterol. The less cholesterol released into the blood stream, the smaller the chance of a blocked artery. One drawback to these older types of statin drugs is that they also decrease CoQ10 and can also decrease cognitive function.

Crestor is also a statin drug, a type of medication known as an HMG-CoA reductase inhibitor. HMG-CoA reductase is a body enzyme that facilitates the production of cholesterol. By inhibiting this enzyme, Crestor causes a reduction in the amount of LDL cholesterol that's produced, resulting in a lower level. LDL cholesterol is considered to be the "bad" type that can lead to heart attacks and other health problems. The use of Crestor also leads to higher levels of HDL cholesterol, considered to be a healthy, beneficial type. Crestor tends to work well, because it is prescribed in higher doses, and so LDL cholesterol can be lowered significantly.

*Both Lipitor and Crestor have a number of cautions associated with them, including for those aged 70 or older without underlying heart disease or those with high blood pressure or diabetes. These cautions include increased risk of developing diabetes and cognition problems (Libov, 2013).*

## Common Steps to Combat High Blood Pressure

Problems with blood pressure are also a reflection of increased inflammation in the body over time and thus, blood pressure medication is widely used to regulate it. Typically, the use of blood pressure-reducing medications will follow the application of cholesterol reducing medication. Although, depending on the state of the patient, both may be started at the same time. You may recall that high blood pressure, obesity and heightened blood sugar levels is part of metabolic syndrome, which increases the risk of heart attack. A few common medications to combat high blood pressure are:

### ACE Inhibitor Class

Basically ACE inhibitors block or help reduce the production of angiotensin-converting enzyme. This angiotensin-converting enzyme narrows blood vessels, and thereby raises blood pressure. So ACE inhibitors help arteries and veins to relax and widen, which then lowers blood pressure.

Lisinopril is a drug of the angiotensin-converting enzyme (ACE) inhibitor class, primarily used in treatment of hypertension, congestive heart failure and heart attacks, and also in preventing renal and retinal complications of diabetes. Again, these ACE Inhibitors help arteries to relax and widen, which then lowers blood pressure. Its indications, contraindications and side effects are as those for all ACE inhibitors— which include cough, dizziness, headache abnormal taste or rash. One nice feature of Lisonpril is that it is not metabolized by the liver and therefore does not cause a toxic buildup of unwanted chemicals in this vital organ.

IrDA, CoIrda, CoAprovel, Karvezide, Avalide and Avapro HCT are all members of another class of blood pressure drugs, but they work on the same principle as above—basically allowing the arteries to relax and widen, therefore lowering blood pressure. They are popular for use in the treatment of hypertension, as reflected in the roughly $1.3 billion in annual sales.

## Beta-blockers and Others

Beta-blockers target the beta receptors, which are found on cells of the heart muscles, smooth muscles, airways, arteries, kidneys, and other tissues that are part of the sympathetic nervous system. Beta-blockers interfere with the binding epinephrine receptors and other stress hormones, and weaken their effect. Side effects of beta-blockers include some risk of diabetes over time (which the ACE inhibitors do not have and can actually help decrease over time) and the heightening of inflammation in the body.

## Alzheimer's Medications

As I have mentioned earlier, there is no known cure for Alzheimer's. However, there are drugs designed to slow the progression of the disease. There are two main types of Alzheimer's medications:

1.  **Cholinesterase inhibitors**
2.  **Memantine**

These medications work in two different brain-messaging systems.

Cholinesterase inhibitors are a type of drug that boosts the amount of acetylcholine (a neurotransmitter) available to nerve cells by preventing its breakdown and elimination in the brain. The end result is that acetylcholine helps to stimulate cognitive function, at least for awhile, until more brain cells die off and there is less net acetylcholine. Aricept, Razadyne, and Exelon (as in "the patch") are a common form of these cholinesterase inhibitors.

Memantine is in a class of medications called NMDA receptor antagonists. It works by decreasing abnormal activity in the brain, and protecting the nerve cells from glutamate, also a neurotransmitter, which is released in excess by Alzheimer's sufferers. Memantine can help people with Alzheimer's disease think more clearly and perform daily activities more easily, but it is not a cure and does not stop the progression of the disease. Namenda is a common name for the drug. Cautions are given with the use of these medications, as some dietary and drug interactions and side effects can be serious—for example, dizziness, confusion, depression, and aggression.

**A Comment Not to be Ignored:**
*Remember, the goal of these Alzheimer's medications is to, in some way, prolong brain function and cognition. However, if brain degradation caused by inflammation and immune system dysfunction is still rampant, the brain will progressively lose the network and resources necessary to function normally.*

## Medications Used for Depression, Agitation and Other Alzheimer's-related Issues

Additional complements to the Alzheimer's medications we've just discussed can be found in the area of antidepressants, antipsychotic and behavior modification drugs. (It seems worthy to note that many times it is a psychologist or psychiatrist who refers a patient to another healthcare professional, who sees beyond the person's most obvious symptoms (e.g., depression) and *then* makes the diagnosis of dementia or Alzheimer's.)

In residential situations, where agitation takes up the time of staff to manage an upset or disruptive patient, these drugs, at least in the past, have been seen as an option to keep a patient compliant and under control. In professional literature, such behaviors as wandering, hoarding, repetitive questioning and other "inappropriate behaviors" may be deemed indications for pharmaceutical drug intervention, depending on the institution. However, some of these drugs have been overused, presumably to 'manage' patients, whether they're behaving inappropriately or not. Hopefully, instances of this practice will die off sooner than later.

**Here are some typical antidepressants:**

Zoloft: Part of a class called tricyclic antidepressants (TCAs). It can be used for the treatment of major depression and obsessive-compulsive disorder (OCD). Side effects may include: liver damage, high blood sugar and diabetes. Although these side effects are rare, they can be a significant consideration with our dementia population.

Celexa: In a class of drugs called selective serotonin reuptake inhibitors (SSRI). It works by increasing the production of serotonin in the body. Celexa can be used for anxiety and panic disorder, and seems to have some positive effect on treating agitation. There are some potential unwanted side effects with this drug, as well however, including slightly decreased mental function and abnormal heart function (Lyketsos 2014).

In addition, here are some pharmaceutical options currently being used for so-called "acting out" or potentially aggressive behavior:

Risperdal: A potent drug that acts as a dopamine antagonist, meaning it reduces the production of dopamine in the body. It is used in the treatment of schizophrenia and treatment-resistant depression. Side effects may include the development of diabetes and increased risk of death in patients with dementia.

Olanzapine (Zyprexa, etc.): Can be used in the treatment of generalized anxiety and panic disorder. Like Risperdal, there are potentially fatal side effects of stroke and death with older patients, and those with dementia-related psychosis have been advised not to use this drug—although, at least in some countries, this advice was being ignored. Global revenues currently stand at $4.4 billion.

Quetiapine (Seroquel, etc.): Also used as a major antidepressant. This was once used in the treatment of Alzheimer's for agitation, and as such, constituted 29% of this drug's total sales. Currently, it is not recommended, as it worsens cognitive function in those with Alzheimer's.

Aritiprazole: This is a second-generation dopamine antagonist that also, like Risperdal, reduces production of dopamine in the body and is used in the treatment of major depression. It is interesting to note that a number of these drugs are also used in the treatment of agitation in children with autism. This drug is not indicated in the treatment for dementia and Alzheimer's, but it is one of the drugs listed as a potential resource. Its side effects include deepening depression, and it is not typically approved for use with adults with dementia.

Clozapine: A very potent antipsychotic drug, typically used as a last resort, due to the possibility of strong side effects such as stroke, fast/irregular heartbeat, heart failure and pneumonia when used by older adults with dementia. Again, as in the case of Aritiprazole (mentioned above), Clozapine is not typically approved for treatment for dementia-related behaviors. Why do I mention it at all in this case? It turns out (see my summary below) that in the past, this drug was used in the treatment of Alzheimer's and dementia.

Haloperidol: Classified as a neurolepic drug, in times past it was considered to be indispensable in the treatment of psychiatric emergency situations. Studies concluded that when administered to Alzheimer's patients with mild behavioral problems, it often made their condition worse. I mention this drug because it is familiar to some of my students who have seen it in use in care facilities for seniors.

**Review and Use of Behavioral Modification Drugs**

Given the possible risks and side effects of these and other drugs used with seniors having Alzheimer's or dementia, it is interesting to note that in a review of the literature (N. Hughes, C.M. and Lapane, K.L. (2005), the conclusion is that, at best, there is only a marginal improvement in behavioral problems. Really, what this points to is how, over roughly the last 20 years, there's been a shift away from these types of drugs being as commonly prescribed to the Alzheimer's population—for the simple fact that they're sometimes *completely* inappropriate. One of the key reasons I bring this to your attention is because of the stories told to me by nursing home employees familiar with current and not-so-current practices in the administration of these drugs. In essence, a growing body of evidence shows the risks outweighing the rewards, and occasionally, in some cases, the appearance of the opposite effects of the drug's intended treatment.

Additionally, the review mentioned above recommended exploration and use of alternative and more noninvasive ways of approaching behavioral modification. Another way of viewing this is: these are quality of care issues, which the cited study addresses. The reviewers suggest that caregiver, patient and family education, as well as various other alternatives, may have a favorable impact on not just quality of care, but the quality of life of those with dementia and Alzheimer's. Our assessment is there *are* other noninvasive ways of addressing agitation and inappropriate behaviors, *with* an accompanying potential for an enhanced quality of life (e.g., better memory function, improved cardiovascular health and social interaction). These are results we've seen using the BodyEnergy Longevity Prescription, and what we'd like to see achieved for all those seniors living with Alzheimer's and dementia.

There is however, one practical downside to this suggestion: it takes more time to manage agitation and dementia behaviors in a non-pharmaceutical way, at least initially. This puts our proposed alternative approach in contrast to the traditional way of approaching the treatment of Alzheimer's patients. Some of this is a question of efficiency, and one can see the dynamics of how this works—it takes 30 seconds to administer a pill to a patient, while in our model, it may take 10–15 minutes *per person* to administer a treatment, and *three to four weeks* to begin to see the change. I believe the broader view of "what is most desirable, in the long run" needs to be taken into consideration, inclusive of what is in the patient's best interest.

Currently, insurance companies and Medicare and Medicaid reimburse for drug treatment, and the time it takes for the administration of such. I can foresee, as I hope you can as well, the time when this new model—the BodyEnergy Longevity Prescription—is recognized as an overall cost-effective, results-oriented non-drug therapy, with both its administration and its reimbursement being integrated into this facet of the healthcare system.

## The Liver

Many of the drugs listed above, especially cholesterol-reducing and antipsychotic drugs, can affect liver function in a negative way. This is why warnings about past or current liver disease and recommendations for periodic liver monitoring are included. The liver is a key organ in the process of digestion and purification of toxic substances from the body. If modifying liver function is a key aspect of how a drug targets an enzyme or processes other substances metabolized by this organ, over time this could essentially compromise and/or shut down liver function, which is necessary to the function of life.

## The Missing Pieces

Central to drug management is the accurate targeting of one symptom or condition at a time. From a biochemical point of view, drugs target very specific enzymes, molecules or processes to create a desired effect. Over time, however, various organs can be pushed beyond capacity, including the liver (mentioned above), the kidneys, spleen, pancreas or heart, to name a few. It seems essential to note, if symptoms are the target and the underlying cause is not addressed, then over time the body's organs can lose their capacity to function in an integrated and balanced manner.

There are two *other* factors that can add to the problems of drug management. First, multiple medications and their interactions with each other can have a deleterious effect. In the list of medications discussed in this chapter, for example, if one has an Alzheimer's condition, certain high blood pressure medications, anti-anxiety and anti-cholesterol treatments may not mix well together. Thankfully, a watchful relative or the new generation of geriatric care managers can sometimes spot potentially harmful drug combinations and take the necessary precautions. And second, aging patients and their organs have seen a lifetime of use, and often cannot tolerate ongoing administration of substances that target one symptom at a time. This is not to say we do not want to treat them, but the potential long-term effects of these drugs in an elderly patient's body must also be taken into account.

## Consequences of the Pharmaceutical Approach

I liken the above approach to managing a houseful of three unruly children. One child who is acting out is put into a corner for a "time out." Another child is very quiet and doesn't get the attention he deserves, because the other children are better at communicating their needs. Yet another keeps disappearing from time to time and is hard to keep track of. Then there are the parents, who are trying to properly run this "three-ring circus." At some point, they may get overwhelmed and have a meltdown themselves. In this analogy, the organs are like the children and the parents are like the body. If no one is coordinating or has the energy for everyone to speak to each other and to the whole, chances are chaos will remain and be the order of the day. I believe there is a better way, or at least a way to integrate other resources within the traditional approach. The next chapter explores some of these options and resources.

Chapter **14**

# Alternative Approaches and Resources

In this chapter, I will switch gears a bit and consider more of the alternative—both preventative and noninvasive—approaches to treating Alzheimer's and dementia. Some of the following may seem obvious, but they are nevertheless valuable resources for caretakers of those with Alzheimer's and dementia, those who may be at risk (even at a much earlier age), and those older seniors who are in the thick of things, as well. My experience in Moscow working with talented neurologists and osteopaths taught me to think of health care using a multigenerational approach, where one generation can inform and take care of the next.

## Functional Medicine

Quite frankly, I had not heard the phrase "functional medicine" until I started actively researching information for this book. The concept of functional medicine was pioneered by Dr. Jeffrey Bland in 1991, soon after which he and his wife Susan founded the Institute for Functional Medicine (IFM). Dr. Bland's work has garnered him many awards, including the Linus Pauling Functional Medicine Lifetime Achievement Award for his outstanding contributions to the field. Other distinguished doctors, such as Dr. Mark Hyman, have played a key role in promoting the influence of functional medicine across the US.

Here are some key principles of functional medicine:

- An understanding of and respect for the biochemical individuality of each human being, based on the concepts of genetic and environmental uniqueness.
- Acknowledgment of the evidence that supports a patient-centered, rather than a disease-centered, approach to treatment.
- Strive for a dynamic balance between the internal and external, the body, mind, spirit and environment
- Familiarity with the web-like interconnections of internal physiological factors.
- Identification of health as a positive vitality—not merely the absence of disease—emphasizing those factors that encourage the enhancement of a vigorous physiology.
- Promotion of organ reserve as the means to enhance the health span—not just the life span—of each patient.

Needless to say, being a craniosacral therapist, I love the modality I practice day in and day out. And I consider functional medicine completely in line with and complimentary to CST principles.

The principle of the biochemical individuality of each human being also certainly rings a bell for those of us in the CST world. Imagine how profound and satisfying it is to actually listen to the deep inner core, or inner physician, of a patient and have that resource tell us what the body needs biochemically. I must say, it is really this experience, of tuning into and following the guidance of the innate healing mechanisms within each patient that has been the teacher for me in all of the work I do...and this book is a reflection of that. I deeply appreciate there have been so many "little and big professors," the countless children and adults I have worked on, who have helped teach me how the body functions and how each person is a truly incredible individual.

One of the things I really appreciate about functional medicine is that it also integrates objective biochemical testing with treatment and listening to the patient's body, and how that body functions as an interrelated unit.

Functional medicine is different from the traditional medical approach, because it reflects an understanding of the origins, prevention and treatment of complex, chronic disease. Hallmarks of a functional medicine approach include:

*Patient-centered care.* The focus of functional medicine is on patient-centered care, promoting health as a positive vitality, beyond just the absence of disease. By listening to the patient and learning his or her story, the practitioner brings the patient into the discovery process and tailors treatments that address the individual's unique needs.

*Integrative, science-based healthcare approach.* Functional medicine practitioners look "upstream" to consider the complex web of interactions in the patient's history, physiology, and lifestyle that could lead to illness. The unique genetic makeup of each patient is considered, along with both internal (mind, body, and spirit) and external (physical and social environment) factors that affect total functioning.

*Integrating best medical practices.* Functional medicine integrates traditional Western medical practices with what is sometimes considered "alternative" or "integrative" medicine, creating a focus on prevention through nutrition, diet, and exercise; use of the latest laboratory testing and other diagnostic techniques; and prescribed combinations of drugs and/or botanical medicines, supplements, therapeutic diets, detoxification programs, or stress-management techniques.

Let's bring to mind, for a moment, the metaphor of "putting out the forest fire" of inflammation in the brain to reduce the symptoms and causes of Alzheimer's and dementia. Steps 6 and 7 of Phase 2, putting out the blaze, involves having an attending physician's support and gathering blood work to verify that changes in diet are having a positive and documentable effect. I will discuss in the next chapter some of the possible benefits to a senior population that can arise from partnering with the Institute of Functional Medicine (IFM) and their talented doctors to monitor positive changes in diet and the degree of inflammation.

## Diet and Nutrition

One of the cornerstones of the functional medicine approach is look-ing at food as medicine. In the past decade, research results in the field of nutrition have given rise to a great deal of discussion about the negative and less than life-supporting effects of various foods and their long-term effects on one's health. This includes information for those like myself, who have spent decades living without regard for the accumulated effects of carbohydrates, sugars and saturated fats. In the following section, I will present three different approaches to diet, nutrition and healing, in order to give you an idea of the benefits that can be derived from each. Just as I mentioned in my comments about functioning recovery and Tami Goldstein, CST, in Chapter 12, one size does not necessarily fit all. The following are suggestions that can be a starting point to explore the possibility of positive change in the health and quality of life for those living with Alzheimer's and dementia.

### The Paleo Diet

Developed by Loren Cordain, Ph.D, the Paleo Diet is based upon the fundamental concept that the optimal diet is the one to which we are genetically adapted. It emphasizes eating protein and vegetables with (as many functional medicine doctors recommend) various supple-ments to bolster and help repair the damage to tissues that may have occurred over long-time exposure to high blood-sugar levels and insu-lin resistance. I have used this diet myself and found this approach fairly easy to implement, even with a busy travel schedule that leans on restaurant fare. (Fortunately, I've noticed many restaurants have become much more flexible and accommodating to the diet requests of their patrons.) The therapeutic effect of the Paleo Diet is supported by both randomized controlled human trials and real-life success stories. The Paleo Diet claims to help produce the following benefits:

- Reduce the risk of heart disease, type 2 diabetes, and most chronic degenerative diseases affecting people in the Western world
- Weight loss, if you are overweight
- Improved athletic performance
- Slow or reverse the progression of autoimmune disease
- Improve or eliminate acne

- Better sleep and more energy throughout the day
- Increased libido
- Improved mental outlook and clarity
- Longer, healthier, more active life

More information can be found by going to: *www.thepaleodiet.com*.

## Mercola Diet

Dr. Joseph Mercola is a pioneering osteopath who considers the following factors in assessing a person's dietary needs:

- Insulin levels
- Weight
- Blood pressure
- Cholesterol levels

According to Dr. Mercola, these are four time-tested, clinically proven "gauges" you can use to determine your own level of health. Indeed, we have previously discussed the above four factors in terms of their being key drivers in metabolic syndrome and the major role they play in the formation of inflammatory processes in the body over time. Dr. Mercola's approach emphasizes the following:

Step 1: Eliminate all wheat, gluten and highly allergenic foods from your diet

Step 2: At least one-third of your food should be uncooked

Step 3: Eat more vegetables

Step 4: Keep your vegetables fresh

Step 5: Limiting sugar and fructose is crucial

Step 6: Avoid artificial sweeteners

Step 7: Avoid situations and foods that contribute to low blood sugar and can lead to hypoglycemia

Step 8: Learn to distinguish physical food cravings from emotional food cravings; where necessary, use info as bridge into getting emotional support and/or counseling

For more information go to: *www.mercola.com/nutritionplan/ beginner.htm*.

## The Dr. Ornish Spectrum

Dr. Ornish, in his book, *Eat More, Weigh Less,* incorporates four elements into a much-heralded heart-healthy" program, three of which

do not include food. He emphasizes the importance of stress management, exercise and "love and support," in addition to nutrition, to bring
about a rejuvenated, more well-conditioned heart and improved overall health. And, he counsels that we will find success, not by restricting
calories, but by "watching" the calories we eat ("When I eat mindfully,
I have more pleasure with fewer calories."). The word "diet" is one he
does not like to use, as he feels his approach is about educating people
in how to make better choices. No food is completely banned in this
approach. He just suggests being mindful about how much we eat of
whatever it is we choose to eat. Dr. Ornish breaks this approach down
into five spectrums, which are basically different degrees of choosing
what is most healthful to least healthful. Eating more from the first few
groups and less from the last few will provide healthier nutritional
food choices.

*Group 1 Foods—Most Healthful:*
Mostly fruits, vegetables, whole grains, legumes, soy products,
nonfat dairy, egg whites (natural form) and good fats that contain
omega 3 fatty acids.

*Group 2 Foods—More Healthful:*
Also mostly plant-based, but can be somewhat higher in monoun-
saturated and polyunsaturated fats. These can include avocados,
seeds and nuts. Small amounts of these types of oils can also be
used. Foods canned in water, canned vegetables (low in sodium),
low-fat dairy are also part of this group.

*Group 3 Foods—Intermediate:*
This group can include seafood and, in moderation, refined carbohydrates and concentrated sweeteners; also, some oils that are
higher in saturated fat, some 2% dairy products, trans-fat-free mar-
garine, sweeteners containing high fructose corn syrup, and higher
sodium amounts than found in Groups 1 & 2.

*Group 4 Foods—Less Healthful:*
Foods that contain additional fat, such as poultry, fish (with higher
mercury), whole milk or dairy products, mayonnaise, doughnuts,
fried rice, pastries, cakes, cookies and pies.

*Group 5 Foods—Least Healthful:*
These foods have the highest trans-fatty acids and saturated fat, including red meat, egg yolks, fried poultry, fried fish, hot dogs, organ meat, butter, cream and tropical oils.

These guidelines are designed for healthy eating. However, if you are looking at reversing heart disease, he recommends some modifications that include limiting fat, cholesterol, caffeine, animal products, sodium, sugar, alcohol and soy products.

Dr. Ornish suggests eating a lot of little meals versus three "normal"-sized meals, because the latter makes you feel hungry more often. By following his recommendations, you will typically feel full faster, and you'll eat more food without increasing the number of calories Dr. Ornish's regimen is more than mere diet. He is an advocate of incorporating at least 30 minutes of moderate exercise a day, or an hour three times a week. He also recommends finding a stress-management technique you can regularly incorporate into your lifestyle, which might include meditation, massage, psychotherapy, or yoga. And finally, he says, having loving support is essential to long-term health. For more information go to: *www.pmri.org/dean_ornish.html*.

## Some Comments on the Above

If you take a careful look at the three approaches outlined above, you'll find some commonalities and some disagreements. For example, the Paleo Diet says "yes" to proteins, including meat, but in most cases avoids legumes. The Mercola Diet recommends that at least one third of a person's food be uncooked. The Ornish Spectrum approach, in its strictest form (i.e., when used for reversal of heart disease), avoids anything with high fat content (meats of all kinds, as well as avocados, nuts and seeds). *What is common to all three is that they are aware of the damaging effects of obesity, high insulin levels, high blood pressure, excessive (if any) sugar intake, gluten and wheat products, and the cumulative effect of foods that cause an initial and ongoing inflammatory response in the body.* Here we see medical professionals embracing the concept that food can have both a negative and positive effect on the overall health and well-being of the body, *and* they all recommend positive steps of action to address and even reverse long-term damage in the body. Indeed, as Hippocrates once said, "Let your food be your medicine, and your medicine be your food."

It is important to note that in addition to diet or nutrition management, many of these health regimen developers emphasize—especially in the case of Dr. Ornish—the importance of exercise and stress management or an integrated lifestyle change. We'll now touch on some further suggestions for these approaches.

**Recommendation on Spices and Fruits**

Here are some great ideas from Dr. Marwan Sabbagh and Beau MacMillan in their wonderful book, *The Alzheimer's Prevention Cookbook: Recipes to Boost Brain Health* (2012):

- Curcumin (Curcuma longa): a potent antioxidant that has been shown to turn off a protein responsible for promoting an abnormal inflammatory response, and also has been demonstrated to lower cholesterol and block formation of amyloid plaques in rats (Barrkowski, 2010).
- Tumeric-curcumin: the active ingredient in turmeric, recommended by Dr. Andrew Weil
- Cinnamon: helps regulate out metabolism and keep our insulin levels in check; also assists in the reduction the accumulation of neurofibrillary tangles
- Blueberries: a subset of polyphenols, which have anti-inflammatory qualities
- Strawberries: same as blueberries, *and* seem to support lowering of oxidative stress

**Supplements**

As part of the healing process of the body, supplements can assist us in filling in the gaps to reinforce our physiology, as our bodies change with age, as well as help us to regenerate at a cellular level, when neglect has taken place. The idea held by many is that vital trace minerals and other substances can allow the cellular environment to more easily find a way to return to its natural structure and function. The key here, as in our previous discussions of how damage can not only be arrested, but also reversed, is that when the body has what it needs, most often from naturally occurring substances, it will automatically respond in a positive way. Here's a short list of supplements, especially those that may be helpful in preventing Alzheimer's and dementia:

- CoQ10
- Alphalimpoic acid

The above are two of the favorite choices of both Dr. John Upledger and Dr. Mark Hyman.

- In addition to the above:
- Coconut oil or coconut milk
- Folic acids/folates
- Especially anti oxidative nutrients such as Vitamin C & E.

## Exercise

Many health authorities have stated that 30 minutes of regular exercise is a key deterrent to the onset of Alzheimer's, in and of itself. There are countless anecdotes of people, many of whom are advanced in years, who have made significant recoveries from Alzheimer's just by getting the body in motion. In Chapter 9, we mentioned the Blue Zones—an innovative program that found "the secrets of aging" by interviewing centenarians. As part of the Power 9 (or nine common practices found in 'blue zone' communities where people live significantly longer *and* better than average), daily exercise is common to all of them. With that said, one of my favorite discoveries is a gentle addition to normal body movement, even if one is confined to a wheelchair: the ancient practice of tai chi, and a variation of the form called tai chi chih. When you behold a room full of eighty-year-olds gently moving in a graceful way, without effort, strain or exertion, and see the glow on their faces, it makes quite an impression. If you are curious and would like to know more, go to *www.taichiforseniorsvideo.com* (Mark Johnson) or for tai chi chih, go to *www.taichichih.org/the-teachers*.

The BodyEnergy Institute is currently reviewing and evaluating programs we can offer in home care, assisted living or nursing home situations, any of which could be modified to the specific needs of seniors.

**CranioSacral Therapy**

Needless to say, craniosacral therapy is highly recommended as a resource for both prevention and treatment of Alzheimer's and dementia. Regular craniosacral therapy increases fluid flow in the brain and is an excellent preventative measure to prevent the buildup of amyloid plaques and tangles in the brain, which further fuel the process of inflammation, autoimmune reaction and eventually brain death. I highly recommend monthly treatment with CST for any of those in an at-risk for Alzheimer's profile, and much more frequently (as discussed in Chapters 11 and 12) for those living with Alzheimer's.

For more information, go to www.BodyEnergy.net to contact our national network of therapists trained to treat the senior population. Also, for more information about the wide variety of non-senior and general programs on CST, go to *www.upledger.com.*

**Meditation and Yoga**

There are five main types of meditation:

- mindfulness
- spiritual
- focused
- movement
- mantra

Within each of these five types of meditation are a myriad of specific meditation techniques. Some of these you may be familiar with are: yoga, Qi gong, guided visualizations, sweat lodges, shamanic rituals, and Healing from the Core (*www.healingfromthecore.com*).

In my own journey for well-being, I have explored Transcendental Meditation. I use this as an example in reference to holistic homeostasis, because it is what I am most familiar with. However, you may find yourself more comfortable using a different approach. As part of an integrated system of lifestyle change and stress management, here are some recommendations:

**Transcendental Meditation (TM)**

As a practitioner of TM for over 40 years, I can attest to the efficacy of this technique, which is easily learned and commonly practiced for 20 minutes, twice a day (morning and evening). Those of you who are a bit older may remember when the Beatles traveled to India to attend a training session at the ashram of Maharishi Mahesh Yogi, the founder of the TM technique. However you may not know that TM is one of the most widely researched self-development techniques in the world today, with over 600 scientific studies performed over the last 30 years.

According to the American Heart Association (AHA), the Transcendental Meditation technique is the only meditation practice that has been shown to lower blood pressure. According to the AHA, "Because of many negative studies or mixed results and a paucity of available trials, all other meditation techniques (including MBSR) received a 'Class III, no benefit, Level of Evidence C' recommendation. Thus, other meditation techniques are not recommended in clinical practice to lower BP at this time."[3] The AHA scientific statement also reported the finding that lower blood pressure through Transcendental Meditation practice is associated with substantially reduced rates of death, heart attack and stroke. The AHA report concludes that alternative treatments that include the Transcendental Meditation technique are recommended for consideration in treatment plans for all individuals with blood pressure > 120/80 mm Hg.

Also, I would like to mention one other aspect of the benefits of stress reduction brought about by the regular practice of TM. It turns out that, besides the beneficial effects of the proper diet in reducing inflammatory processes in the body, there are hormones such as homocystine that reflect just how well the body reacts to stress in the environment. Higher levels of these hormones also may cause higher levels of inflammation in the body and form the basis for autoimmune disease to be exhibited. The practice of TM has a beneficial effect in regulating these stress hormones and bringing increased noninflammatory balance to the body, thereby providing a preventative resource to all those who practice it.

For more information, go to *www.BodyEnergy.net/TM* client program or *www.TM.org*.

---

[3] Brook R.D., et al., Beyond Medications and Diet: Alternative Approaches to Lowering Blood Pressure. A Scientific Statement from the American Heart Association. *Hypertension*, 61:00, 2013.

**Yoga**

Here I am distinguishing "yoga" from meditation, in the sense that yoga—whose origin can be found described in the ancient classical texts of India—is a gentle form of stretching that builds both strength and flexibility in the body, and can be modified to meet the needs of a widely varying population. Practicing yoga is also a useful way of supporting continued flexibility in the body, which indirectly helps support increased cardiovascular and cerebrospinal fluid (CSF) flow, and is thereby a preventative measure to help offset Alzheimer's and dementia.

Just like meditation techniques, there are many forms of yoga to explore. One of the many resources comes from the Harvard University Center for Wellness: *www.agelessyoga.org/yoga_for_seniors.html*.

Here, we have really just 'scratched the surface,' in terms of the available resources that are both preventative and regenerative in nature. For more information and continued updates on these and other resources for ongoing health and recovery support, please go to: *www.BodyEnergyinstitute.org*.

## Chapter 15

# A Call to Action

Working in the healthcare field for many years, I've observed that if you're a senior and don't have an advocate, or someone on your side, especially when you get sick (especially if you're afflicted with Alzheimer's and dementia), you are basically 'up the creek,' without anyone reviewing what the healthcare system is doing for *or* to you.

Therefore, I will begin this final chapter with a few stories I think illustrate just how vulnerable to Alzheimer's and medical/pharmaceutical intervention our senior population is, and the importance of family and friends in supporting them throughout the stages of this process. In addition, I hope you'll be able to see in these anecdotal stories the pivotal role of our institutional structures, especially regarding how we *currently* address those with Alzheimer's and dementia, *and* what changes can be made to enhance the treatment and quality of life of all those afflicted by these diseases—including bringing the BodyEnergy Longevity Prescription into increasingly more widespread use by the medical professionals who deal with Alzheimer's and dementia.

Indeed, this chapter is about the interaction between institutions, both public and private, regarding the treatment and ongoing care of people living with Alzheimer's and dementia—throughout all stages of this process (prevention, at risk, early, middle and late stages)—and the importance of letting our voices be heard about precisely how this support is currently working. We all have varying degrees of trust in the people and communities that support our loved ones. Some of us have been raised to have unquestioning acceptance of the kind of treatments, the type of care, and the type of procedures that are offered to our parents as they age. On the other end of the spectrum, there are those who are skeptical of what may be offered to us, our children, and our parents. Most people's stance is likely somewhere in the middle. My intention in writing this book is to offer information that can give a broader perspective on what has become the norm and strike more of a balance for the good of all. This is not the first time a call for change and a different way of looking at treating a disease process has happened in the history of healthcare and social support and services. I believe we all have the right to ask whatever questions we need to in order to have the most accurate, far-reaching view of what we can do about Alzheimer's *and* get the answers we deserve. In a very real sense, we are the customers of the healthcare and senior care system. This being so, we can formulate the conditions for our satisfaction and state the outcomes we expect from those who provide for us.

## Mary Ann's Mom

When my friend Mary Ann's mother began exhibiting some early signs of dementia about a year ago, she felt, somewhat painfully, it was time to help her make the move to an assisted living facility (ALF). She did so, and after about a year of living there, her mom began showing indications of high blood pressure, something she'd never had before. Significantly enough, she was being fed a lot of processed food at this particular ALF. Then, her mom had what looked liked signs of a small stroke. The staff did not immediately inform Mary Ann of the stroke, but just offhandedly mentioned it during her next visit. After spending several days in the hospital for observation, Mary Ann's mom was discharged. In the interim, the supplements her mom had received from her daughter were removed from the room. Fortunately, Mary Ann was able to meet with her mother's doctor (the third in a row she had "inherited" after doctor transitions and moves). Mary Ann explained what she saw as the benefits of the supplements and, to her delight, the new doctor welcomed the advice, saw nothing wrong with the supplements, and wrote them into her orders for medication.

The following questions arise in my mind, and I believe all of them are legitimate, reasonable concerns: "When there is not someone committed to monitoring an Alzheimer's patient's status and standing up for their interests, what happens to him or her?" "What happens when you don't have someone around who is willing to take the time to look after you?" "If you're alone and have Alzheimer's, whose advice will you follow...and will it be the right advice?"

Another example of the use or misuse of drug therapy is reflected in a study I mentioned in Chapter 13, a study which reviewed the inappropriate use of psychotropic drugs in nursing homes. The authors' suggested that, at least in some instances, poor prescribing techniques led to overuse or inappropriate use of these psychotropic drugs as a way to 'manage' behavior in a nursing home environment. The study pointed out these types of practices also adversely affected the quality of life of these residents. What initially led me to review these outcomes was a report about the practice of 'overmedicating' dementia patients from one of my students who worked as a senior home nursing assistant in a facility in northern Iowa. It's worthy of noting, many of these patients had no family close by or available for consultation. My student recorded her observations of "problem" (agitated) patients before and after the administration of psychotropic, "behavior management" drugs. Before the administration of the drugs, the patients were agitated, but also able, to some extent, to communicate their needs and frustrations. *After* the administration of these drugs, the patients were basically nonverbal, listless and unable to express any ability to think in any way, shape or manner—that is, their quality of life was significantly diminished.

Our proposal is simply that gentle, noninvasive, hands-on therapy can achieve some measure of reduction of agitation—thereby helping to manage behavior in a positive way—and, at the same time, improve overall cognitive function, social interaction and the ability to better perform some of the activities of daily living, such as self-feeding, brushing of teeth, etc. As has been indicated previously (Chapter 6), in an initial pilot study, when craniosacral therapy was administered to Alzheimer's and dementia patients, these types of positive outcomes were observed, including patients' ability to self-feed, improvement of communication, and some degree of cognitive and memory improvement. In this example, we are simply pointing out that other options may be available, that result in much better outcomes.

## A Hopefully Inspiring, If Not Thought-Provoking Conversation About Senior Healthcare Standards

What these stories have in common is that there was an intervention, admittedly non-medical, to assist seniors with Alzheimer's and/or dementia. It really points to the need for more input and assistance by caregivers and relatives. Remember, 75% of seniors with Alzheimer's or dementia are treated by internists or general medical practitioners, as opposed to the pediatric population, where 75% of children see a pediatrician. This is not so much a criticism of the medical community; rather, it demonstrates there has been a lack of specialization in senior care, especially regarding those with Alzheimer's and dementia. Certainly, there are many reasons for such a lack of specialization, perhaps the primary ones being driven by economic incentives (after all, seniors typically can afford less for treatment). Cultural factors can have an effect, as well. Nevertheless, the needs and characteristics of seniors are different from those of the general population, just as children and infants are different from adults. To *not* take into account the unique needs and differences in an aging population, *including* psychological differences, is to miss the ever-emerging gap between the general population and the 80+ million Baby Boomer population.

Having said this, I see two key factors setting the stage for a discussion of how things could be different for senior care: economics and "quality of life."

## Economics

One of the drivers of change, I predict, will be the ever-increasing costs of senior healthcare over the next 20 years. As I have discussed previously, we do have an emerging health crisis in the US, and it is starting decades before the general population reaches its 60th year. Here is the picture in broad brush strokes: there are currently 25 million people diagnosed with diabetes, 7 million more undiagnosed, and an estimated 80 million who are pre-diabetic. That totals over 100 million people, or roughly a third of the US population. A certain percentage of those folks will develop cardiovascular disease, say anywhere from 20-30%. That would translate into 20-30 million. Now a certain percentage of this group of 100 million, not necessarily even having cardiovascular challenges, will develop the symptoms of Alzheimer's and dementia— perhaps 10-15 million over the next 20 years (according to current estimates, the number of cases doubles every 20 years). However, this is not a frozen figure. It is estimated over the next 20 years that in the general US population, the incidence of diabetes and pre-diabetes will be one in two of the general population. So the percentage of "down the line" symptoms like cardiovascular disease or Alzheimer's and dementia may change (that is, increase) this figure, as well.

It is important to state that just because someone is pre-diabetic doesn't mean they will become diabetic. Or if someone is diabetic, it doesn't mean they will develop cardiovascular problems. Or if someone has cardiovascular problems or diabetes, they will develop Alzheimer's or dementia. *However,* there is enough evidence to support saying there is a good likelihood of these happening. Remember, many doctors refer to Alzheimer's as type 3 diabetes. And we know at least anecdotally that 40% of people in an Alzheimer's unit have some form of diabetes. So there is enough data to lead to the conclusion that diabetes and Alzheimer's are connected. As we have discussed, this is over and above other factors that contribute to inflammatory processes in the body that raise the overall number of "down the line" cases of dementia and Alzheimer's we have pointed to.

What does all this have to do with economics, especially on a national scale? This may be where public, private and corporate interests are in a state of conflict, to put it mildly. I have discussed in Chapter 9 some of the main "drivers" of the current health care system that create profit for the private sector: prescription drugs and diet-related factors. The current way to approach diseases such as Alzheimer's and cardiovascular problems is to address or suppress the symptoms. Neither of these get at the root causes of these problems. Over several decades, this treatment approach may manage the symptoms, but

eventually the more serious "end stages" of these diseases will manifest, and the public cost—in terms of loss of productivity, increased
pressure on caregivers (either paid or not) and the overall public burden on taxpayers—is a significantly weighty consequence no one can
or should ignore. In that sense, it is an overall public burden that all of
us will be responsible for, and disproportionately so for the younger
generations.

We have also discussed how the food available to us may contribute to inflammation in the body. One could ask, "If there is a suspected
link between these two, why doesn't the food industry change what
it offers to the public?" One would think, if tens of millions of people
display symptoms of obesity, pre-diabetes and full-blown diabetes,
the general population must be getting something—food-wise—
that does not lead to optimal health. Of course, there is more to the
story. Once someone develops diabetes or is at risk for cardiovascular
disease, they are encouraged to take drugs to moderate their blood
pressure, cholesterol, and other factors. Very often, once on a regimen of drugs, they will keep taking them to control the symptoms.
At $50–200 a month for medication, multiplied by millions of people,
this becomes an attractive ongoing source of cash revenues. The direct
beneficiaries of these ongoing cash revenues are the pharmaceutical
companies. There is, however, one other piece to the puzzle. The professionals who prescribe these medications are the doctors or medical
community who employ a spectrum of tests and drugs to combat the
symptoms. One could almost say there is a synergy between all three
groups: the largest food producers, the pharmaceutical companies
and the medical professionals dispensing the drugs. Some might feel
it is just a coincidence, but one can't help but wonder and speculate if
there is more to it.

Of course, the obvious answer is that motivation for profit may
drive a lot of this. On the other side of this equation is the cost to the
public and even every individual taxpayer, let alone the direct cost to
seniors. If 20–40 million people or more over a period of time develop
any of these symptoms, who will take care of them, especially as they
age? As we have seen in public debates, most probably it will fall on the
shoulders of the younger generation. Here we have not addressed the
direct and indirect social costs, which are estimated to run anywhere

from $2–20 trillion dollars by 2050, much of which will be borne by the public and public services, to some extent?

At some point then, I am suggesting public and private interests may reach an impasse. One scenario is to cut taxes, privatize health-care, eliminate the Medicare and Medicaid budget and let everyone fend for themselves. However, there is another outcome I would like to suggest. As medical technology and healthcare costs increase, per-haps at some point it will force policymakers to take a closer look at non-traditional options, including manual therapies such as CST, and the effectiveness of a healthy, alternative diet. Someone may come to the conclusion that these approaches are, in fact, much less expensive, noninvasive, and can deliver better results. Studies would, of course, have to demonstrate the effectiveness of alternative approaches, but I am confident that if the economic pressure becomes great enough, some amazing discoveries will be made.

Please know that I do not suggest this naively. Not all of this will happen easily. Still, I am committed to providing those who are at risk or who have Alzheimer's with the best possible alternatives to choose from, to heal whatever damage has been done and reverse the effects of the disease.

In summary, there doesn't have to be a conflict between private industry and the welfare of the public. Ask the CEO of Safeway stores, Steve Burd, who, as was mentioned previously, instituted a program to reward healthy lifestyle choices and cut over $100 million annually in healthcare costs. As he said, "Making money and doing something good are not mutually exclusive." In other words, a win-win solution is possible with enough public education and encouragement by us, the customers of the food and healthcare system.

## Quality of Life for Those in Senior Care

Economics and quality of life intertwine. As we have seen, the type of treatment a senior receives is often reflected in the attitudes of those who treat them. In our chapter, "Going Against the Grain," we explored how current attitudes may influence what is thought to be possible as our seniors age. Let me explain this a bit more. Most people would agree they don't mind aging if they are well and healthy—it's the discomfort and decline they don't like.

The current paradigm is that aging and decline are inevitable. It may not be stated out loud, but the assumption is there. After all, we see it all around us. In senior care facilities, there is a formula of sorts, encompassing everything from the food that is served, the types of activity provided, the doctors who are available and the drugs that are commonly prescribed. This formula seems, in a sense, to be derived from the old industrial mass production model (perfect for adapting to the incoming Baby Boomer generation), relatively easily adapted to senior living, where meals are served, oftentimes, to hundreds of residents at a time, a range of 'senior activities' are made available, and the typical medical interventions and drug treatments are standardized. After all, it makes sense to create a model to process millions of people more efficiently, from a corporate point of view. A doctor specializing in geriatrics may see things in the same way (or perhaps differently). Those specializing in geriatrics (and many new doctors will be trained in the coming years) have the option to continue sustaining the "decline is inevitable" paradigm, or on the other hand, these same doctors can choose to change the way we think about aging, and begin to look at aging as a change of physiology where more long-term health, longevity and sustained quality of life are possible.

Within this culture is also a sub-conversation about "quality of life," meaning just how well the residents (or their children) like how they are being treated and how comfortable they feel. Of course, when we are discussing Alzheimer's and dementia, the topic of this conversation is even more relevant, with specialized rules and procedures to manage the quality of life of a more medically fragile population. All of this reflects the best efforts of many (often understaffed and overworked) dedicated employees.

All of this has led me to formulate two new concepts: The Senior Alternative Bill of Rights, and the notion of "Being a Customer of the Senior Healthcare System." Here is a way to start looking at what we can expect as far as treatment and care, *and* what to ask for.

# Senior Alternative Healthcare Bill of Rights

1. The right to alternative therapy.
2. The right to a healthy diet
3. The right to exercise and freedom of movement.
4. The right to non-drug alternatives
5. The right to enhanced quality of life
6. The right to clear explanations of expected outcomes
7. The right to accessibility to friends, family and community
8. The right to have private pay treatment.
9. The right to dignity, respect and a place in society as an elder.
10. The right for a physician to say 'I don't know'
11. The right for an elder to choose their own time of transition.

## Comments on the Senior Alternative Healthcare Bill of Rights:

1. **The Right to Alternative Therapy.** This is simply a way of saying that alternative therapies such as CST may offer stabilization of a condition and even improvement over time. If a therapy is noninvasive and practiced with care and respect, simple hands-on skills may be much more cost-effective *and* include the human connection and listening that is known to be part of the healing process.

2. **The Right to a Healthy Diet.** As Dr. Karyn Shanks, who I recently interviewed for a DVD production, observed, "The diet and nutrition offered to seniors on an institutional basis could stand some improvement. Even simple changes in the amount of sugar and inflammatory foods one eats could make a significant difference." (Watch *Your Health, The Nation, and the Senior Healthcare System* or go to www.BodyEnergy. net for more information).

3. **The Right to Exercise and Freedom of Movement.** Many of our seniors have lived healthy lifestyles and remain active. However, once at a senior care or assisted living facility, many (certainly not all) may be restricted in their movement, sometimes just because of the distances from one part of the facility to another. A simple exercise program, even for those wheelchair-bound, should be made available as part of their in-residence process.

**4.    The Right to Non-Drug Alternatives.** This is also part of the changing landscape of the senior care industry. I believe that drug therapy should be used with consideration and reflection, and that doctors serve their patients best when they are looking at causes, not just symptoms. Admittedly, this takes more time and analysis, but this is part of the process of promoting "conscious aging," no matter where our loved ones are located. Often there are other, non-drug options for healing that address conditions that may have been developing over long periods of time.

**5.    The Right to Enhanced Quality of Life.** The concept here is that the way we look at aging can be altered, no matter where a senior lives. Central to this belief is the idea that vitality and well-being can actually improve *and not decline* as age increases. Of course, inherent in this observation is the idea that additional resources may make a difference in how well-being is maintained.

**6.    The Right to Clear Explanations of Expected Outcomes.** This "right" is as much for the caregivers and children as for residents in a facility. My own experience is there are often underlying assumptions about the outcome of treating a chronic or acute disease process. I believe we have the right to know what a healthcare professional is thinking, even if it is what we might not want to hear. At least, then, we have a feeling for where the treatment is headed and can make decisions about how that meets our expectations or desires. We can then entertain other options, as well.

**7.    The Right to Accessibility to Friends, Family and Community.** A "right" to having access to loved ones and the community ties into some of the previous comments about quality of life. It is my observation that diet, non-drug alternatives and other complementary therapies result in more conscious and alert aging, giving the person a greater sense of control and a more positive, healthier attitude. This "result" is a two-way street. When relatives and friends see their loved ones are more present, their visits and interactions are richer and the healing process builds on itself. Mainly, this "right" is about accessing the power of love or connectedness.

**8.    The Right to Have Private Pay Treatment.** This is, in most cases, a non-issue. If family members want to provide supplemental treatment, it should be considered or allowed, as long as it is not disruptive to other aspects of the facility. Currently, certain treatments or modalities are officially practiced to the exclusion of all else, even though other approaches may offer more encouraging results. My goal is to include what might now be considered "private pay" as part of the standard list of services.

**9. The Right to Dignity, Respect and a Place in Society as an Elder.** This is really a cultural comment. When I interviewed Dr. Bill Thomas, he stated, "The Baby Boomer generation is redefining what elderhood means and will have a significant effect on how this looks in society." Taking the broad view, every culture has had a different way they respect and look to their elders for counsel and advice. As Simon de Bouvier observed, "The way a culture treats their elders is a reflection of the quality of that civilization."

**10. The Right to Choose One's Own Time of Transition.** This really is a statement about conscious aging, as much as it is available. I've observed that the more a patient has access to their own "inner process," the easier it is for them, on some level, to know when to transition to the next phase of their existence, regardless of their belief system. There are a variety of ways in which this "choice of experience" can be played out. Certainly, when a loved one passes away surrounded by friends and family, it is an altogether different scenario than when someone passes away alone. The type of modalities I have been discussing in this book, such as CST, promote a listening that makes it easier for a senior at this stage of life to be attuned to their inner process and know when, at least in many circumstances, it is the right time to "let go." Our elders deserve such dignity and respect.

## Being a Customer of the Senior Healthcare System

Now that I've suggested a senior's bill of rights, the next concept revolves around how to become a wiser, more satisfied customer of the healthcare system. Simply put, we have the right to ask for what we want, and to ask questions of those who provide products and services for our well-being and that of anyone we know with Alzheimer's. Quite frankly, consumers have power and they shape what is and can be offered to them.

Here is a brief bit of history to support this concept. I remember, quite by chance, looking at an article in *USA Today* in the 1990's that stated over 50% of healthcare customers were going to massage therapists and other similar modalities (like CST) and paying cash for their treatments. Not long after, the Office of Alternative Medicine was formed by the medical community to study the effects of these alternative procedures. For a time, Dr. Upledger was on the board of directors of this organization. I suspect the organization was formed to look at why these alternative practices were so popular, and why in the world customers would pay out-of-pocket for such procedures. After all, a great deal of medical practice is based on insurance, and out-of-pocket costs are, at least in many cases, minimal.

I think the reason this statistic was as high as it was (and likely still is) is that a great many people found, and still find, these procedures to be effective. One could imagine this could be viewed as a sort of competitive challenge by "the powers that be," much in the same way certain organizations have attempted to regulate various supplements, including vitamins.

My view on all of the above is to look at the evidence and ask the question, "What procedure or practice produces the best outcome and quality of life, no matter where it comes from?" Of course, a follow-up response to this question could be to look at the experience of Dr. Dean Ornish, whose "heart healthy" program was finally endorsed and covered by Medicare *after 16 years.* His view is that once something alternative is endorsed and embraced by the traditional community, it has a significantly positive impact. Public acceptance and reimbursement signals a "sea change," a change in the way culture views what is possible. In other words, when presented with someone who has Alzheimer's, I am saying (and looking to both the general public and the medical community at large to embrace the worthiness of this approach) that the BodyEnergy Longevity Prescription offers a reasonable set of practices and procedures to improve the quality of life and potentially halt and even reverse the effects of the disease.

Now, I am not waiting for Medicare reimbursement for many of the procedures and suggestions we are making in the BodyEnergy Longevity Prescription. However, as the old saying goes, "The more attention we bring to something, the more it grows"—and here, the faster the change occurs. This principle can actually be applied to the concept of "a call to action": in this case, we're beginning by asking those who are 50+ and living with Alzheimer's (or a family member or a loved one or an attending doctor) for consideration of the BodyEnergy Longevity Prescription, then inclusion in the patient's protocol, then (at first) by private pay, eventually by insurance reimbursement (likely finding it less costly than current traditional procedures), and ultimately by Medicare and Medicaid, such that all citizens with Alzheimer's will enjoy the maximum benefit.

Integrating the concepts we have discussed in this book, what I am proposing next are a series of questions that are worthy of asking either your senior healthcare manager or your parent's (or your loved one's) healthcare provider, as well as some proposed healthcare standards to most effectively support both ourselves and our aging population.

## Questions for Your Senior Healthcare Manager

1. How do you feel about diet at your facility?
2. Do you understand the relationship between food, inflammation and diabetes?
3. Have you heard that some researchers are calling Alzheimer's Stage 3 diabetes? And why do you think they say that?
4. Are you open to allowing alternative therapists to treat patients at your facility?
5. Are you willing to allow your PT's, OT's and speech therapist to learn new techniques that may be of assistance to patients in your facility?
6. Are you willing to consider the above to be covered under existing billing guidelines? Or on a private pay basis?
7. How you do define "quality of life" for your residents?
8. What is the long-term goal you have for supporting your residents?
9. Do you believe senior health improves or declines over time? Why?

It is important to remember the context for most doctors seeing Alzheimer's patients is that they are general practitioners or
internists, not geriatric specialists. So the questions below are, at
the very least, meant to educate them, as much as they are meant to
assist you in understanding their background and ability to support
your loved ones.

## Questions for Your Parent's or Loved One's Healthcare Provider

1.  I believe there is a connection between diet, inflammation and dia-
    betes in relation to Alzheimer's. What can you tell me about that?
2.  Have you heard that some researchers are calling Alzheimer's type
    3 diabetes? What are your thoughts on that?
3.  What would you prescribe for the treatment of Alzheimer's and
    dementia? Why?
4.  I am interested in complementary care for my loved one. I have
    read that craniosacral therapy could be beneficial. Have you heard
    of it?
5.  The reason why I am interested in craniosacral therapy is I under-
    stand that the flow of craniosacral fluid decreases with age, and
    that it is often as much as 75% less in patients with senile demen-
    tia. I think that this therapy could help. What do you think?
6.  How do you feel about non-pharmaceutical interventions? Are you
    open to looking at supplements that may augment the diet and
    intake of my loved one?
7.  Do you believe that a senior's health can improve, or does it only
    decline?

The above questions are primarily meant to stimulate conversation
and give you some gauge about how open your healthcare provider and
facility provider might be. My standard is, the more open, the better.

## A Different Approach: Green House Homes

Here is an example of senior care with a twist. Dr. Bill Thomas, founder of the Eden Alternative, a philosophy and program that, over the last 20 years, de-institutionalized nursing homes in all 50 states, gave a great TED talk titled, *Elder-hood Rising: The Dawn of a New World Age* (*www.changingaging.com*). In his TED talk, Dr. Thomas points out how it is possible to create senior living facility where the elder is honored and has a place to speak, be heard, and to be taken care of in an individualized manner. And very recently, National Public Radio (NPR) filed a report on Mr. Thomas' efforts to transform the nursing home industry. His "Green House Homes" concept, totaling 148 homes nationwide, represents approximately 1% of the total nursing home community in the US. I believe he is an inspiring spearhead of change, and it is in alignment with what we are attempting to do: improve the health and quality of life of those living with Alzheimer's as much as possible.

Ina Jaffe, who filed the report for NPR, describes what many of us envision when we think of nursing homes: sharing a room with a stranger, people slumped over in wheelchairs, bad smells. She points out that Dr. Thomas feels the current nursing home concept is outdated. After all, many of the homes were designed in the 60's and 70's and are nearing the end of their useful life. Dr. Thomas' own reflection as a gerontologist is, that in many cases, he was prescribing medications for seniors who are, at core, combating loneliness. So he thought, *What is next?* His thoughtful response to that question is how the Green Homes concept emerged: an emphasis on smaller facilities, with an average of 12 residents per facility, with individual rooms and bathrooms, the capacity for encouraging mobility without the use of wheelchairs, *and* a flexible eating schedule. What is most encouraging is that the cost to fund such a facility falls into the median cost of existing senior healthcare around the country. This is perhaps, one of the most inspiring new models of senior care *with* the potential to integrate CST, functional medicine, non-inflammatory diets, and other progressive ideas into their programs. (See Dr. Thomas also on our new DVD documentary, *Your Health, the Nation, and the Senior Healthcare System.*)

## It's Time, Now, For a Call to Action

So all of this now leads to some "action steps" tailored to each segment of the population. Being realistic and not knowing how far we are from a fundamental shift in our national/international perspective, we need full participation from everyone to reach our goal. The following are suggestions, gleaned from all we have discussed up to this point.

## For Seniors aged 60–90+: Preventative Maintenance.

*Quality of Life for the Rest of Us, the 'Young Old'*

My definition of "quality of life" is a bit different. It would incorporate the assumption that aging and longevity can be maintained for an extended period of time, with the elder having the inner resources to be tuned into themselves and to know when they are at the end of their life cycle. In my "CranioSacral Therapy for Longevity; Reversal of the Aging Process" class, I explore how various techniques can help enhance the vitality of each person and increase the gap between their chronological and biological age. The greater the gap, the more resource they have to draw upon. At the other end of the spectrum, when we look at the more medically complex clients, those who have been diagnosed with a variety of what I call "the diseases of aging," and may be on multiple medications. This would include Alzheimer's and dementia.

Here, then, is the quality of life spectrum we can observe in the aging process for those between 60 and 90+ years old: at the one end, those who remain young and vital during these years, and at the other, those who suffer from chronic and debilitating disease. Anyone in this age spectrum could have the same chronological age, but a very different quality of life. Based on my own observation and clinical experience, it is assumed that, with the proper support, the "young old" as Mary Piepher puts it, or healthy senior, *can* maintain their well-being for an extended period of time. However, the other major assumption I make is that the "old old" can actually arrest their decline, stabilize their condition, and even improve their health. Evidence of this thinking is not in great supply, but it is there. I mentioned "Blue Zones" back in Chapter 9—they are areas in the world where seniors have managed to live long and with a good quality of life. I believe the model of the Blue Zones has a potential for being duplicated in this modern, fast-moving culture, as well. I mentioned in Chapter 10 ten steps for prevention, as well as further "action steps" to extend the possibility of remaining in the 'young old' category.

As I have mentioned previously, an ounce of prevention is worth a pound of cure. Again, we can characterize this population as the "young old." Most of us in the Baby Boomer generation want to stay young and vibrant for as long as possible and we are, in a sense, redefining the concept of aging. As the saying goes, "Sixty is the new fifty." But of course, a lot of us may feel our age more than others. Here are some suggestions, which echo our suggestions in Chapter 10, to maintain our youth and well-being:

1. *Diet.* Certainly, we'll highly recommend that your diet is non-inflammatory in nature. It would be quite useful to see if any insulin resistance is present, as well as any other markers in the blood that signal potential problems. Based on that analysis, one could tailor a diet that would best serve a "young old" senior's needs (refer to the appendix for a variety of nutrition and diet resources).

2. *Meditation and stress management.* Based on an assessment of the stress levels in one's life, meditation and some form of simple yoga or stretching may be useful. It is not just your diet that can lead to inflammation, but stress as well, as indicated by the stress hormones in the blood. My personal choice to combat ongoing and accumulated stress is the Transcendental Meditation (TM) program, which I have practiced for over 40 years. For more information, go to my website *www.BodyEnergy.net*, and look under meditation and stress management. Also, take a look in the appendix of this book for a list of other stress management resources.

3. *Craniosacral Therapy.* As my mentor, Dr. John Upledger, used to say, "Craniosacral therapy is motion producing therapy." Simply put, the more fluid our bodies are, the less creaky and stiff we become. I recommend a treatment every one or two months, just to maintain health and help prevent any of the diseases of aging from forming in the system. You may go to the Upledger website, *www.upledger. com/findapractitioner* or *www.BodyEnergy.net*, to find a therapist near you.

4. *Functional Medicine.* For information about how to address any long-term health problems noninvasively, go to the Institute of Functional Medicine (IFM) website to find a local practitioner (*www.functionalmedicine.org*).

5. *Exercise.* Exercise has been shown to be a valuable part of an ongoing healthy lifestyle. Whether it be tai chi or any of the more traditional forms of exercise (such as walking), exercise is an ideal preventative practice. Look in our appendix for more exercise resources.

## For Caregivers at Home

It is oftentimes a challenge for caregivers living at home to take care of themselves *and* the needs of a loved one with Alzheimer's, but there is an increasing network of resources geared toward those who take care of those with Alzheimer's at home. In addition to the suggestions mentioned above, I would suggest looking into our 2-day classes, "CranioSacral Therapy for Longevity: Applications for the Treatment of Alzheimer's and Dementia (CSLAD)," which are designed for laypersons and therapists working in senior care. Go to *http://BodyEnergy. net/services-2#2day* to find a list of local classes offered, or contact me via the website to discuss the opportunity of bringing the class to your area. In addition, the American Alzheimer's Association and Maria Shriver's website offer resources for caregiver support.

## For Therapists in Assisted Living, Nursing Homes and Memory Care Facilities, as well as CNA's, RN's, LMT's, PT's, OT's and Speech Therapists.

The 2-day class, "CranioSacral Therapy for Longevity: Applications for the Treatment of Alzheimer's and Dementia" (CSLAD) described above offers valuable and easily learned craniosacral therapy (CST) skills that can be integrated and applied in a professional setting. Additionally, the CSLAD is qualified to offer CEU's or educational credit for continuing education, including recent certification by the American Speech Therapy Association (ASHA). Ask your nursing home administrator to see if such accreditation is available for your specific profession and if they would be willing to consider such training as an adjunct to services offered at your faculty. In addition to the training aspect, there is of course the treatment aspect. Ideally, in the scope of services that can be reimbursed during the course of your treatment, CST could be included, which would make it even more accessible to a wider variety of residents. The BodyEnergy Institute welcomes your partnership in creating a dialogue to include such services as part of your scope of practice. To that end, the BodyEnergy Institute has created a case history template available at *www.BodyEnergy.net* to help you document your treatment progress and add to our growing database.

## For Nursing Home Administrators

The BodyEnergy Institute has created an information package that is available for you, in order for you to evaluate how our program can be integrated into your facility. I am currently conducting beta site evaluations at various locations across the country to document the effectiveness of our program. Besides the gathering of case history reports mentioned above, I welcome your participation in finding ways to use our program to enhance quality of life measures for your residents, whether in a single location or multiple venues. We also invite you to investigate and monitor how our programs may assist in managing agitation of residents in your facility with decreased medication. My focus is to help add to a growing body of evidence-based medicine that can offer healthy, positive options to your clients.

Additionally, there is a growing network of trained certified senior craniosacral therapists who are available to make on-site visits to administer our techniques. As another option, CST training can be offered in house to your staff. As well as offering training for your staff, I am currently seeking to have CST treatment covered as an additional billable treatment modality by your resident's insurers. In the interim, the BodyEnergy Institute would like to partner with you to create options for private pay treatment by your residents on an individual basis, and/or include this program as part of an enhancement available to residents facility-wide. I realize the industry has competition in offering services and quality of life enhancements, and wish to help all nursing home administrators be at the cutting edge in a changing marketplace.

## For Craniosacral Therapists

Those of you who have completed the Upledger Institute's SER1 (or above) are in a unique position to assist in the growth of our specialization in the senior population. Just as many of you have specialized and taken Upledger Institute classes in pediatrics, the "Longevity" curriculum gives you the tools to assist this growing segment of the population and participate in the programs outlined above. I invite you to look at our training in CSLAD and CSLRAP, and consider becoming a part of the growing national network of trained CST therapists providing services to seniors, as described above. As our program matures, we are also looking for trained therapists to become part of multi-hand therapy teams to address all aspects of diseases of aging, with the goal of maintaining well-being and health for the entire senior population.

## For Public Policymakers

Obviously, there are many pressures upon those of you who are elected officials who have made a wholehearted commitment to serve the public. I wish to propose a balance in the area of senior healthcare between "for profit" private industry and the needs of the public. Those of you who formulate public policy are well aware of rising healthcare costs, the growing number of our older citizens, and the economic burden—which is increasing over time—of supporting a population that is unwell. You are in a unique position to examine the evidence and find ways to both protect the general population *and* minimize direct and indirect economic costs to the US population and economy over the next 30 years. This can be a win-win situation, with support of both the private and public insurance industry and the Medicare and Medicaid system. If the complementary approaches discussed in this book are made available to a larger segment of the senior population and incorporated into what is currently practiced, our belief is that the incidence of chronic disease, including Alzheimer's and dementia, can and will be diminished. Quite frankly, something different than what has been done and is currently being done must be considered to avert a growing national healthcare crisis. We invite your participation and that of all public policymakers in helping to change the healthcare system from an illness-based approach to one based on wellness.

## For Adult Children of Parents Living with Alzheimer's

As a caregiver concerned about giving the best possible support to your parents, you are one of the most important people for whom I'm writing. Indeed, this book is about providing both education and resources to help in your decision-making process. I realize a great deal of information presented here may be new to you, but it is based on years of observation and experience, not just by me, but by thousands of craniosacral therapists nationwide and around the world. We invite you to look into our CSLAD training program for laypersons and consider how even a few simple changes may make a difference. Use the questions outlined above, if you like, to open a dialogue with your parents' healthcare professionals and senior care facility administrators. These questions are offered as a resource to expand the conversation about how best to support your parents in getting the health care and quality of life they so truly deserve.

## A Final Thought

This book, ultimately, is a passionate plea for change. We've seen how our investigations reflect a growing health crisis in the US *and* worldwide. Alzheimer's and dementia are really at the tip of an often silent iceberg, with the "acknowledged conditions" quietly fueled by improper diet (or at the very least, a lack of healthy alternatives), environmental toxicity and lack of public education. We've also reviewed the consequences of not properly addressing the direct and indirect costs of healthcare for an aging, more vulnerable population. However, it is not just the senior population's healthcare we must currently manage better *and* plan for more wisely. The younger generation's lives and lifestyles are also exhibiting conditions that currently have *and* in the future will continue to have a significant economic impact on the healthcare system. Extrapolate this impact to 10–20 years from now and the direct care costs, left unattended, will also proportionately increase into a similar crisis situation.

In addition, we must reflect on the indirect costs, which are reflected in the burden passed on to all of us, and the consequent impact on our national creativity, spirit and productivity. Here, we are focusing on the economics of the matter, but as the children, parents and caregivers of our loved ones, we have a stake in the outcome of this healthcare system crisis, as well. A plea for change encourages *all* of us to consider the alternatives we *know* are less invasive and cost neutral, if not altogether less costly.

As most CST practitioners know, our techniques do not necessarily stand alone and therefore may not be the only therapeutic modality we use. Many of us have continually kept ourselves open to and diligently studied and practiced other modalities that we've recognized can maximize the repair, recovery and rejuvenation for patients of all ages. Our intention has always been (and continues to be) to stack the cards in favor of our clients and loved ones.

As the saying goes, "The ball is now in your court." Use the information provided in this book to explore, reflect and, wherever necessary, do your own research. My hope is that you will be inspired to begin taking action to make the BodyEnergy Longevity Prescription (or at the very least, a regular routine of craniosacral therapy treatments) available to your loved one(s), your patients, your residents or the citizens whom you serve. We have done our best to provide you with a solid foundation from which you can take a great stride forward, to significantly enhance the health, well-being and quality of life of those living with Alzheimer's and dementia. May this book's offerings serve you well.

*Our most sincere intention is captured in the words of Dr. John Upledger: "We want to help people."*

If you would like to know more about the concepts discussed in this book, or join a longevity support group in your area, go to *www.bodyenergy.net/longevitysupportgroup*

# REFERENCES

## Chapter 1

Alzheimer's Association. "Inside the Brain: An Interactive Tour."
  *www.alz.org/braintour* (2014)

Centers for Disease Control and Prevention. "Leading Causes of Death."
  *http:/www.cdc.gov/nchs/fastats/lcod.htm* (2013)

Alzheimer's Association. "Alzheimer's Disease Facts and Figures."
  *http:/www.alz.org/alzheimers_disease_facts_and_figures.asp* (2014)

Wimo, Anders. "The World Alzheimer Report 2010: The Global Economic
  Impact of Dementia." Martin Institute of Psychiatry, King's College,
  London, UK. *www.alz.org/documents/national/world_alzheimer_report*
  (2010)

Cummings, Jeffrey. "Jeffrey Cummings on Early Diagnosis for Alzheimer's."
  *http:/www.archive.sciencewatch.com/ana/st/alz2/11augSTAlz2Cumm*
  (2011)

Shrestha, Laura B. and  Heisler, Elayne J. "The Changing Demographic
  Profile of the United States." Congressional Research Service.
  *www.fas.org/sgp/crs/misc/RL32701.pdf* (2011)

Gerdner, L., et al. "Craniosacral StillPoint Technique: Exploring Its Effects
  in Individuals with Dementia." Journal of Gerotological Nursing.
  Vol 34. (2008)

Best, Ben. "Alzheimer's Disease: Molecular Mechanism."
  *www.benbest.com/lifeext/Alzheimer.htm* (2014)

Centers for Disease Control and Prevention. "Heart Disease."
  *www.cdc.gov/nchs/fastats/heart.htm* (2012)

Ornish, Dean 'Yes Prevention is Cheaper than Treatment' Preventative
  Medicine Research Institute  *http:/www.pmri.org/research.htm* (2008)

Davis, William. Wheat Belly: Lose the Wheat, Lose the Weight and Find
  Your Path Back to Health. HarperCollins Publishers Ltd., Canada (2012)

Centers for Disease Control and Prevention. "Press Release," October 22, 2010. *http://www.cdc.gov/media/pressrel/2010/r101022.html* (2010)

Upledger, John E. "The Expanding Role of CerebralSpinal Fluid in Health and Disease." *http://www.massagetoday.com/mpacms/mt/article.php?id=10426* (2002)

AARP Foundation. *http://www.assets.aarp.org/external_sites/caregiving/index.html* (2014)

## Chapter 2

Best, Ben "Alzheimer's Disease: Molecular Mechanisms." *http://www.ben-best.com/lifeext/Alzheimer.html* (2014)

Selkoe, Dennis "Cell Biology of the Amyloid beta-Protein Precursor and the Mechanism of Alzheimer's Disease" [Abstract]. Annual Reviews, A Non Profit Scientific Publisher. *http://www.annualreviews.org/doi/abs/10.1146/annurev.cb.10.110194.002105?journalCode=cellbio.1* (1994)

Morris, John. "Special Topic of Detecting Alzheimer's at the Preclinical Stage." *www.archive.sciencewatch.com/ana/st/alz2/11octSTAlz2Morr/* (2011)

Cummings, Jeffrey."Jeffry Cummings on Early Diagnosis for Alzheimer's" *http://www.archive.sciencewatch.com/ana/st/alz2/11augSTAlz2Cumm* (2011)

Mattson, Mark "Mark Mattson Discusses the Relationship Between Energy Metabolism and Alzheimer's." National Institute of Aging. *www.archive.sciencewatch.com/ana/st/alz2/11julSTAlz2Matt/* (2011)

Selkoe, Dennis. "Dennis Selko on The Amyloid Hypothesis of Alzheimer's Disease." *http://www.archive.sciencewatch.com/ana/st/alz2/11marSTAlz2Selk/* (2011)

Perry, George. "George Perry on the Role of Oxidative Stress in Alzheimer's Disease." *http://www.archive.sciencewatch.com/ana/st/alz2/11junSTAlz2Perr* (2011)

Bennett, David. "David Bennet on Identifying Risk Factors for Alzheimer's" *http://www.archive.sciencewatch.com/ana/st/alz2/11sepSTAlz2Benn/* (2011)

Snowdon, DA "Healthy aging and dementia: findings from the Nun Study" [Abstract]. NCBI *http://www.ncbi.nlm.nih.gov/pubmed/12965975* (2003)

Whitney, Howell. "Amyloid imaging the next frontier." Diagnostic Imaging. com *www.diagnosticimaging.com/amyloid-imaging-next-frontier-alzheimer%E2%80%99s-care* (2012)

Combs, Colin K., Johnson, Derrick E. Karlo J. Colleen, Cannady, Steven B., Landreth, Gary E. "Inflammatory Mechanism in Alzheimer's Disease: Inhibition of β-Amyloid-Stimulated Proinflammatory Responses and Neurotoxicity by PPARγ Agonists" [Abstract]. The Journal of Neuroscience *http:/www.jneurosci.org/content/20/2/558.short* (2000)

American Journal of Psychiatry "Inflammatory mechanisms in Alzheimer's disease-implications for therapy." (abstract) *www.ajp.psychiatryonline.org/article.aspx?articleID=170489* (1994)

Akiyama H et al NCBI. "Inflammation and Alzheimer's Disease." NCBI *www.ncbi.nlm.nih.gov/pmc/articles/PMC3887148/* (2000)

Trojanowski, John Q., Y. Lee, Virginia M. "Fatal Attractions of Proteins: A Comprehensive Hypothetical Mechanism Underlying Alzheimer's Disease and Other Neurodegenerative Disorders." *www.onlinelibrary.wiley.com/doi/10.1111/j.1749* (2006)

Wolfe, Michael S., De Los Angeles, Joseph, Miller, Duane D., Xia, Weiming, Selkoe, Dennis J. "Are Presenilins Intramembrane-Cleaving Proteases? Implications for the Molecular Mechanism of Alzheimer's Disease." *http:/www.pubs.acs.org/doi/abs/10.1021/bi991080q* (1999)

Journal of Alzheimer's Disease "Top 100 Most Prolific Alzheimer's Researchers." *www.j-alz.com/top100/Prolific.html* (2014)

Straten, G., Eschweiler, G.W., Maetzler, W., Laske, C., Leyhe. "TGlial Cell-Line Derived Neurotrophic Factor (GDNF) Concentrations in Cerebrospinal Fluid and Serum of Patients with Early Alzheimer's Disease and Normal Controls" Journal of Alzheimer's Disease. *http://www.j-alz.com/issues/18/vol18-2.html Pages 331-337* (2009)

Science Watch. "Special Topic: Alzheimer's Disease Top 20 Authors." *www.archive.sciencewatch.com/ana/st/alz2/authors/* (2011)

Hardy, John. "John Hardy on Genetics-Based Alzheimer's Disease Research." *www.archive.sciencewatch.com/ana/st/alz2/11aprSTAlz2Hard/* (2011)

## Chapter 3

Administration on Aging. "Projected Future Growth of the Older Population." *www.aoa.gov/aoaroot/aging_statistics/future_growth/future_growth.aspx#* (2014)

Siegel, Jacob "Aging into the 21st Century" Administration on Aging (1996)

## Chapter 4

Upledger, John, E. Cell Talk: Talking to Your Cell(f). North Atlantic Books, Berkeley, CA (2003)

"The Expanding Role of CerebralSpinal Fluid in Health and Disease." *www.massagetoday.com/mpacms/mt/article.php?id=10426*

Sutherland, Adah. With Thinking Fingers. Cranial Press (1962)

Upledger, John, E. CranioSacral Therapy: What It Is, How It Works. North Atlantic Books, Berkeley (2008)

James, Gavin, A., and Strokon, Denni. "The Significance of Cranial Factors in Diagnosis and Treatment with the Advanced Lightwire Functional Appliance." *www.alforthodontics.com/Drs%20James%20Strokon%20 03_3%20IJO.pdf* (2003)

Silverberg, G.D., et al. "Assessment of low flow CSF drainage as a treatment for AD: results of a randomized pilot study." Neurology 59(8): 1139 *www.ncbi.nlm.nih.gov/pubmed/12391340* (2002)

Dettmore, Diane, et.al. "Use of Nursing Theory to Guide Clinical Practice." *www.ncbi.nlm.nih.gov/pmc/articles/PMC3365866/* (2009)

Upledger, John, E. A Brain is Born: Exploring the Birth and Development of the Central Nervous System. North Atlantic Books, Berkeley (1996)

## Chapter 5

Devanand, S., et al. "Molecular mechanisms of aging associated inflammation." Cancer Letters (Online international journal). 236.1 13-23. (2006)

Perry, V.H. " The impact of systemic inflammation on brain inflammation." Advances in Neuroscience and Clinical Rehabilitation." Volume 4, Number 3, July/Aug. (2004)

Sompayrac, Lauren M. How the Immune System Works. John Wiley & Sons, Sussex, UK (2012)

Dinarello, C. A. "Proinflammatory cytokines." Chest Journal (2000)

Glabinski, R., et al. "Regulation and Function of central nervous system chemokines" International Journal of Developmental Neuroscience (1995)

Ghimikar, R., et al. "Inflammation in traumatic brain injury: role of cytokines and chemokines" Neurochemical Research (1998)

Susumu, Tonegawa. "The Nobel Prize in Physiology or Medicine 1987: Discovery of the genetic principle for generation of antibody diversity." Wikipedia. *www.en.wikipedia.org/wiki/Susumu_Tonegawa* (2014)

MacMillan, Beau and Sabbagh, Marwan. The Alzheimer's Prevention Cookbook: Recipes to Boost Brain Health. Ten Speed Press, Berkeley, CA (2012)

"The Expanding Role of CerebralSpinal Fluid in Health and Disease." *www.massagetoday.com/mpacms/mt/article.php?id=10426*

# Chapter 6

May, C., Kaye, J.A., Atack, J. R. Schapiro, M.D., Friedland, R.P., & Rapoport, S.I. "Cerebrospinal fluid production is reduced in healthy aging." Neurology 40 (3, pt.1) 500 (1990)

"The Expanding Role of CerebralSpinal Fluid in Health and Disease." *www.massagetoday.com/mpacms/mt/article.php?id=10426*

"Craniosacral StillPoint Technique: Exploring Its Effects in Individuals with Dementia." Journal of Gerotological Nursing. Vol 34. (2008)

Salmon, JH "Senile and Presenile dementia: Ventriculoatrial shunt for symptomatic treatment" Geriatrics 24(12), 67-72. (1969)

Silverberg, G.D., Levinthal, E., Sullivan, E.V., Bloch D.A., Chang, S.D., Leverenz, J. et.al. "Assessment of low-flow CSF drainage as a treatment for AD: Results of randomized pilot study" Neurology 59, 12139-1145 (2002)

Rubenstein, E. "Relationship of senescence of cerebrospinal fluid circulation system to dementia of the aged." Lancet 351, 283 (1998)

Thrane, Vinita Rangroo; Thrane, Alexander S.; Plog, Benjamin A.; Thiyagarajan, Meenakshisundaram; Iliff, Jeffrey J.; Deane, Rashid; Nagelhus, Erlend A.; Nedergaard, Maiken. "Paravascular microcirculation facilitates rapid lipid transport and astrocyte signaling in the brain" Scientific Reports 3 nature.com (2582) *www.nature.com/srep/2013/130904/srep02582/full/srep02582.html* (2013)

Dettmore et al. "Aggression in Persons with Dementia: Use of Nursing Theory to Guide Clinical Practice." NCBI *www.ncbi.nlm.nih.gov/pmc/articles/PMC3365866/* (2009)

Whitney L.J. Howell. "Diagnostic Imaging." *www.diagnosticimaging.com/ amyloid-imaging-next-frontier-alzheimer%E2%80%99s-care* (2012)

Whiley Online Library. "Inverse relation between in vivo amyloid imaging load and cerebrospinal fluid Aβ42 in humans" [Abstract]. www. onlinelibrary.wiley.com/doi/10.1002/ana.20730/abstract (2005)

Felgenhauer, K. "Protein size and cerebrospinal fluid composition." Klin. Wochenschr 52(24): 1158–64. PMID 4456012. (1974)

Saunders, NR., Habgood, MD, Dziegielewska, KM. "Barrier mechanisms in the adult brain." Clin. Exp. Pharmacol. Physiol. 26 (1): 11–9. PMID 10027064. (1999)

Johanson, et.al. "Multiplicity of cerebrospinal fluid functions: New challenges in health and Disease." Cerebrospinal Fluid Res 5(10). *www. ncbi.nlm.nih.gov/pmc/articles/PMC2412840/ /* (2008)

Brown, P.D.; Davies, S.L.; Speake, T., Millar, I.D. "Molecular Mechanisms of Cerebrospinal Fluid Production." *www.ncbi.nlm.nih.gov/pmc/articles/ PMC1890044/* (2004)

## Chapter 7

Whitmer, R.A. "Type 2, Diabetes and Risk of Cognitive Impairment and Dementia." Current Neurology and Neuroscience Reports 7, no. 5: 373 (2007)

Hyman, Mark. The Blood Sugar Solution. Little Brown & Co. (2012)

van Himbergen, Thomas M., PhD; Alexa S. Beiser, PhD; Masumi Ai, MD; Sudha Seshadri, MD; Seiko Otokozawa, MT; Rhoda Au, PhD; Nuntakorn Thongtang, MD; Philip A. Wolf, MD; Ernst J. Schaefer, MD. "Biomarkers for Insulin Resistance and Inflammation and the Risk for All-Cause Dementia and Alzheimer Disease."Journal of the American Medical Association. (2012)

The Alzheimer's Prevention Cookbook: Recipes to Boost Brain Health. Ten Speed Press, Berkeley, CA (2010)

Barberger-Gateau, P., Raffaitin, C., Letenneur, L., Berr, C., Tzourio, C., Dartigues, J.F., Alperovitch, A. "Dietary Patterns and Risk of Dementia: The Three-City Cohort Study." Neurology 69, no. 20: 1921 (2007)

West, R., Schnaider Beeri, M., Schmeidler, J., Hannigan, C.M.Angelo, G., Grossman, H.T., Rosendorff, C. Silverman, J.M. "Better memory functioning associated with higher total and LDL cholesterol levels in very elderly subjects without the APOE4 allele." American Journal of Geriatric Psychiatry. (2008).

King, D.E., Mainous III, A.G., Buchanan, T.A., Pearson, W.S. "C-Reactive Protein and Glycemic Control in Adults With Diabetes." Diabetes Care. (2003)

Tilg, H., Moschen, A.R. "Adipocytokines: Mediators linking adipose tissue, inflammation and immunity." *http://www.nature.com/nri/journal/v6/n10/abs/nri1937.html* (2006)

Administration on Aging. "Projected Future Growth of the Older Population." *www.aoa.gov/aoaroot/aging_statistics/future_growth/future_growth.aspx#* (2014)

Houston, Mark. What Your Doctor May Not Tell You about Heart Disease. Grand Central Life & Style, New York (2012)

Weil, A. "The Depression-Inflammation Connection." *http://www.huffingtonpost.com/andrew-weil-md/* (2011)

Sarkar D and Fisher PB "Molecular mechanisms of aging associated inflammation." Cancer Letters. 236.1: 13-23. *http://www.ncbi.nlm.nih.gov/pubmed/15978720* (2006)

"Metabolic Syndrome." Wikipedia. *http://en.wikipedia.org/wiki/Metabolic_syndrome* (2014)

Whitmer, R.A., et al. "Central Obesity and Increased Risk of Dementia Three Decades Later." Neurology 71, no. 14: 1057 (2008)

Dimopoulos, N., Piperi, C., Salonicioti, A., Psarra, V., Mitsonis, C., Liappas, I., Lea, R.W., and Kalofoutis, A. "Characterization of the Lipid Profile in Dementia and Depression in the Elderly." Journal of Geriatric Psychiatry and Neurology. (2007)

## Chapter **8**

Davis, William. Wheat Belly: Lose the Wheat, Lose the Weight and Find Your Path Back to Health. HarperCollins Publishers Ltd., Canada (2012)

Perlmutter, D., Loberg, K. Grain Brain: The Surprising Truth about Wheat, Carbs, and Sugar — Your Brain's Silent Killers. Little, Brown and Company (2013)

Oz, Mehmet, M.D. "Five-foods-should-never-be-in-your-grocery-cart." *http://www.doctoroz.com/videos* (2010)

Kendall-Tackett, K. The Psychoneuroimmunology of Chronic Diseases: Exploring the Links Between Inflammation, Stress, and Illness. American Psychological Association, Washington, DC (2009)

Energy News. *http://enenews.com/radiation-dose-triples-at-tokyo-monitoring-post-early-sunday-doubles-at-another* (2012)

Goldstein, Tami. Coming Through the Fog. Outskirts Press (2013)

Cave, Stephanie What Your Doctor May Not Tell You About Children's Vaccinations. Warner Books, NY (2001)

Kirby, David. Evidence of Harm. St. Martin's Press, NY (2005)

Dinarello, C. A., "Anti-cytokine therapies in response to systemic infection" Journal of Investigating Dermatological Symptoms and Procedures. (2001)

American Autoimmune Related Diseases Association. "List of Autoimmune and Related Diseases. Research Report." *www.aarda.org/autoimmune-information/list-of-diseases/* (2011)

American Diabetes Association. "Statistics About Diabetes." *www.diabetes.org/diabetes- basics/diabetes-statistics/* (2011)

National Diabetes Education Program. "The Facts About Diabetes: A Leading Cause of Death in the U.S." *ndep.nih.gov/diabetes-facts/* (2014)

Lazarus, R.S., and Folkman, S. "Stress, Appraisal and Coping." Springer Publishing Company (1984)

Selye, Hans. The Stress of Life. McGraw-Hill, New York (1978)

Sheraton, et al. "Researchers see a 'picture' of threat in the brain: Work may lead to a new model of inflammation." *http://researchnews.osu.edu/archive/anxbrain.htm* (2011)

Cohen, Shelton. "Chronic stress, glucocorticoid receptor resistance, inflammation, and disease risk." *http://www.pnas.org/content/109/16/5995* (2012)

Cherry, Olschowka and O'Banion. "Neuroinflammation and M2 microglia: the good, the bad, and the inflamed." *http://www.jneuroinflammation.com/content/11/1/98* (1998)

C. Franceschi, F. Olivieri, F. Marchegiani, M. Cardelli, L. Cavallone, and M. Capri. "Genes involved in immune response/inflammation." *http://www.readcube.com/articles/10.1016/j.mad.2004.08.028* (2005)

"Diabetes mellitus." Wikipedia. *www.en.wikipedia.org/wiki/Diabetes_mellitus* (2011)

Harford, K.A., Reynolds, C.M., McGillicuddy, F.C., and Roche, H.M. "Fats, Inflammation, and Insulin Resistance: Insights to the Role of Macrophage and T-Cell Accumulation in Adipose Tissue." Proceedings of the Nutrition Society 70, no.4: 408 (2011)

Amor, S., Puentes, F., Baker, D., and van der Valk, P. "Inflammation of Neurodegenerative Diseases." Immunology 129, no. 2: 154–69 (2010)

Central Obesity and Increased Risk of Dementia Three Decades Later. Neurology 71, no. 14: 1057–64 (2008)

## Chapter 9

Henke, N., and Kadonaga, S. "Improving Japan's health care system." www.mckinsey.com/insights/health_systems_and_services/improving_japans_health_care_system/ (2009)

Berwick, Don. Escape Fire: Designs for the Future of Health Care. Jossey Bass (2003)

Alazraki, MGlobal. "Pharmaceutical Sales Expected to Rise to $880 Billion in 2011." Daily Finance. http://www.dailyfinance.com/2010/10/07/global-pharmaceutical-sales-expected-to-rise-to-880-billion-in/ (2010)

Brownlee, S. "Will Health Care Reform Make U.S. Healthier?" www.newamerica.net/node/91023 (2013)

Ornish, Dean. "Dr. Dean Ornish on the Oprah show." www.ornishspectrum.com/video/dr-ornish-on-the-oprah-show-part-2-of-3/

Buettner, Dan. The Blue Zones: Lessons for Living Longer From the People Who've Lived the Longest. National Geographic Society (2013)

"Pharmaceutical Industry." Wikipedia. http://en.wikipedia.org/wiki/Pharmaceutical_industry (2013)

World Health Organization. " Essential Medicines and Health Products." Information Portal. http://apps.who.int/medicinedocs/en/d/Js6160e/6.html (2013)

PMRI. Ornish, Dean. "Biographical information." http://www.pmri.org/dean_ornish.html (2014)

## Chapter 10

Piper, Mary. Another Country: Navigating the Emotional Terrain of Our Elders. Berkley Publishing Group (1999)

MacArthur Foundation. "Growing Older But Not Old: Insight on Aging and Health." _http://www.macfound.org/press/publications/growing-older-not-old-insight-aging-and-health/#sthash.r00kJ8qS.dpuf_ (2013)

Pew Research. "Attitudes about Aging: A Global Perspective." http:// _www.pewglobal.org/2014/01/30/attitudes-about-aging-a-global-perspective/_ (2014)

Caspersen, et al. "Mitochondrial Aβ: a potential focal point for neuronal metabolic dysfunction in Alzheimer's disease." The FASEB Journal - Express article 10.1096/fj.05 3735fje (2005)

Hotamisligil. "Mitochondria: Dynamic Organelles in Disease, Aging, and Development."

Nature 444, 860 _www. doi:10.1038/nature05485_ Published online: 13, December 2006

Blackburn, E. "The Roles of Telomeres and Telomerase." _http://www.ibiology.org/ibioseminars/genetics-gene-regulation/elizabeth-blackburn-part-1.html_

Umbdenstoc Richard J. "Opportunities for Collaboration Between Health and Health Care." The Robert Wood Johnson Foundation. _www.rwjf.org/en/blogs/new-public-health/2012/04/richard- j-umbdenstock-american-hospital-association-opportunities-for-collaboration-between-health-and-health-care.html_ ( 2012)

Medicare.gov. "Nursing Homes - Alternatives to Nursing Home Care." _www.medicare.gov/nursing/alternatives.asp_ (2012)

## Chapter 11

Seneff, S., Wainwright, G., Mascitelli, L. "Nutrition and Alzheimer's disease: The detrimental role of a high carbohydrate diet." European Journal of Internal Medicine (2010)

Kang, J.H., Ascherio, A., and Grodstein, F. "Fruit and Vegetable Consumption and Cognitive Decline in Aging Women." Annuals of Neurology 57, no. 5: 713 (2005)

Scarmeas, N., Stern, Y., Mayeux, R., and Luchsinger, J.A. "Mediterranean Diet, Alzheimer Disease, and Vascular Mediation." Archives of Neurology 63, no. 12: 1709 (2006)

Scarmeas, N., Stern, Y., Mayeux, R., Manly, J.J., Schupf, N., and Luchsinger, J.A "Mediterranean Diet and Mild Cognitive Impairment." Archives of Neurology 66, no. 2: 216 (2009)

Feart, C. Samieri, C. et al. "Adherence to a Mediterranean Diet, Cognitive Decline, and Risk of Dementia." Journal of the American Medical Association 302, no. 6: 638 (2009)

Scarmeas et al. "Physical Activity, Diet, and Risk of Alzheimer Disease." Journal of the American Medical Association 302, no. 6: 627—37

Morris, M.C., Evans, D.A., Tangney, C.C., Bienias, J.L., Wilson, R.S. "Association of Vegetable and Fruit Consumption with Age-Related Cognitive Change." Neurology 67, no.8: 1370—6 (2006)

Ford, E.S. "Does exercise reduce inflammation? Physical activity and C-reactive protein among U.S. adults." Epidemiology (2002)

Goldstein, Tami A. Coming Through the Fog. Outskirts Press (2013)

## Chapter 12

Ornish, Dean. "Don't Tread on Me: Transcending the Left/Right Wing Health Care Debate." Huffington Post August 28, 2009

Cherry, Kendra. "Adult Neurogenesis: Can We Grow New Brain Cells?" *http://psychology.about.com/od/biopsychology/f/adult-neurogenesis.htm*

"Paravascular microcirculation facilitates rapid lipid transport and astrocyte signaling in the Brain." Scientific Reports 3 (2582). *www.nature.com/srep/2013/130904/srep02582/full/srep02582.html* (2013).

Rennels M.L., Blaumanis, O.R., Grady, P.A. "Rapid solute transport throughout the brain via paravascular fluid pathways" [Abstract]. Adv Neurol. 52: 431 *www.ncbi.nlm.nih.gov/pubmed/2396537* (1990)

Takano, T., Tian, G.F., Peng, W., Lou, N., Libionka, W., Han, X., Nedergaard, M. "Astrocyte-mediated control of cerebral blood flow." [Abstract]. Nat Neurosci 9 (2): 260 *http://www.ncbi.nlm.nih.gov/pubmed/16388306* (2006)

Somerville, H. "Safeway CEO Steve Burd has legacy as a risk-taker." Mercury News. *http://www.mercurynews.com/ci_23227100/safeway-ceo-steve-burd-has-legacy-risk-taker* (2013)

Perlmutter, David. "Neurogenesis: How to Change Your Brain." Huffington Post *www.huffingtonpost.com/dr-david-perlmutter-md/neurogenesis-what-it-mean_b_777163.html* (2010)

Newport, M. "What if there was a cure for Alzheimer's and no one knew?" Self-Published Case Study (2008)

NCBI. Dooley, N.R. and Hinojosa, J. "Improving Quality of Life for Persons With Alzheimer's Disease and Their Family Caregivers: Brief Occupational Therapy Intervention." *www.ncbi.nlm.nih.gov/pubmed/15481783* (2014)

Cserr, H.F. "Physiology of the choroid plexus." Physiol Rev. 51 (2): 273 *www.ncbi.nlm.nih.gov/pubmed/4930496* (1971)

Rennels, M.L., Gregory, T.F., Blaumanis, O.R., Fujimoto, K., Grady, P.A. "Evidence for a 'paravascular' fluid circulation in the mammalian central nervous system, provided by the rapid distribution of tracer protein throughout the brain from the subarachnoid space." Brain Res. 326 (1): 47 *http://www.ncbi.nlm.nih.gov/pubmed/3971148* (1985)

Ichimura, T., Fraser, P.A., Cserr, H.F. "Distribution of extracellular tracers in perivascular spaces of the rat brain." Brain Res. 545 (1–2):10 *http://www.ncbi.nlm.nih.gov/pubmed/1713524* (1991)

Cserr, H.F., Cooper, D.N., Suri, P.K., Patlak, C.S. "Efflux of radiolabeled polyethylene glycols and albumin from rat brain" [Abstract]. Am J Physiol. 240 (4): F319 *http://www.ncbi.nlm.nih.gov/pubmed/7223889* (1981)

Xie, L., Kang1, H., Xu, Q., Chen, M.J., Liao, Y., Thiyagarajan, M., O''Donne, J., Christensen, D.J., Nicholson, C., Iliff, J.J., Takano, T., Deane, R. Nedergaard, M. "Sleep Drive Metabolite Clearance from the Adult Brain." Science 342 (6156): 373– *http://www.sciencemag.org/content/342/6156/373* (2013)

Mehler, M.F., Gokhan, S. "Mechanisms underlying neural cell death in neurodegenerative diseases: alterations of a developmentally-mediated cellular rheostat." Trends Neurosci. 23 (12): 599 *www.ncbi.nlm.nih.gov/pubmed/11137149* (2000)

Becker, Robert. Body Electric Harper, NY (1998)

Cell Talk: Talking to Your Cell(f). North Atlantic Books, Berkeley, CA (2003).

# Chapter 13

Sonnen, J.A., et al. "Nonsteroidal Anti-Inflammatory Drugs are Associated with Increased Neuritic Plaques." Neurology 75, no. 13: 1203 (2010)

Wilcock, G.K., Ballard, C.G., Cooper, J.A., and Loft, H. "Memantine for agitation/aggression and psychosis in moderately severe to severe Alzheimer's disease: a pooled analysis of 3 studies." *http://www.ncbi.nlm.nih.gov/pubmed/18294023* (2008)

Libov, C. "Be Cautious of Statins If You"re Over 70: Top Heart Doctor."
Newsmax Health October 2013

"Sertraline." Wikipedia. *https://en.wikipedia.org/wiki/Sertraline*

"Citalopram" Wikipedia. *http://en.wikipedia.org/wiki/Citalopram*

"Risperdal" Wikipedia. *http://en.wikipedia.org/wiki/Risperidone*

Preidt, Robert "Celexa May Help Ease Alzheimer's-Linked Agitation" Web
MD *www.webmd.com/alzheimers/news/20140218/antidepressant-cel-exa-may-help-ease-alzheimers-linked-agitation* (2014)

"Olanzapine." Wikipedia. *en.wikipedia.org/wiki/Olanzapine* (2014)

"Haloperidol." Wikipedia. *en.wikipedia.org/wiki/Haloperidol* (2014)

"Quetiapine." Wikipedia. *en.wikipedia.org/wiki/Quetiapine* (2014)

"Aripiprazole." Wikipedia. *en.wikipedia.org/wiki/Aripiprazole* (2014)

"Clozapin." Wikipedia. *en.wikipedia.org/wiki/Clozapin* (2014)

Daiello, L.A. "Atypical antipsychotics for the treatment of dementia-related behaviors: An Update." Pubmed *http://www.ncbi.nlm.nih.gov/pubmed/17633594* (2007)

Hughes, C.M. and Lapane, K.L. "Administrative Initiatives for Reducing
Inappropriate Prescribing of Psychotropic Drugs in Nursing Homes:
How Successful Have They Been?" NCBI *www.ncbi.nlm.nih.gov/pubmed/15839722* (2005)

Mayo Clinic "Diseases and Conditions, Alzheimer's Disease." *www.mayoclinic.org/diseases-conditions/alzheimers-disease/in-depth/alzheimers/art-20048103* (2014)

Cohen-Mansfield, J., Thein, K., Marx, M.S., Dakheel-Ali, M. "What are
the barriers to performing nonpharmacological interventions for
behavioral symptoms in the nursing home?" *www.ncbi.nlm.nih.gov/pubmed/21872537* (2011)

Woodward, M.C. "Pharmacological Treatment Of Challenging Neuro-pychiatric Symptoms of Dementia." Journal of Pharmacy Practice
and Research Volume 35, No. 3. *www.jppr.shpa.org.au/lib/pdf/gt/sept2005.pdf* (2005)

## Chapter 14

Barrkowski, Ann. "Tumeric for Inflammation." *http://www.livestrong.com/article/405988-what-are-the-benefits-of-turmeric-leaves/* (2010)

Dumont, M. Kipiani, K. Yu, F., Wille, E., Katz, M., Calingasan, N.Y., Gouras, G.K., Lin, M.T., and Beal, M.F. "Coenzyme Q10 Decreases Amyloid Pathology and Improves Behavior in a Transgenic Mouse Model of Alzheimer's Disease." National Institute of Health (2012)

Ford, E.S. "Does exercise reduce inflammation? Physical activity and C-reactive protein among U.S. adults." Epidemiology (2002)

Walton, K., Levitsky, D. "Effects of Transcendental Meditation Program on Neuroendocrine Abnormalities Associated with Aggression and Crime." Transcendental Meditation in Criminal Rehabilitation and Crime Prevention. p.67 (2003)

Rosenthal, N.E. Transcendence: Healing and Transformation Through Transcendental Meditation. Penguin Group (2011)

Snow, L.A., Hovanec, L. and Brandt, J. "A Controlled Trial of Aromatherapy for Agitation in Nursing Home Patients with Dementia." The Journal of Alternative and Complementary Medicine,10(3): 431-doi:10.1089/1075553041323696. _http://online.liebertpub.com/doi/ abs/10.1089/1075553041323696_ (2004)

Brook, R.D., et al. "Beyond Medications and Diet: Alternative Approaches to Lowering Blood Pressure: A Scientific Statement from the American Heart Association." Hypertension 61:00. (2013)

Barnard, Neal. Dr. Neal Barnard's Program for Reversing Diabetes. Rodale Press (2007)

Sparks, L.M., et al. "A High-Fat Diet Coordinately Downregulates Genes Required for Mitochondrial Oxidative Phosphorylation in Skeletal Muscle." Diabetes 54: 1926-33 (2005)

Morris, M.C, Evans, D.A., Tangney, C.C., Bienias, J.L., Wilson, R.S., Aggarwal, N.T, and Scherr, P.A. "Relation of the Tocopherol Forms to Incident Alzheimer Disease and to Cognitive Change." The American Journal of Clinical Nutrition 81, no. 2 508 (2005)

Pocernich, C.B., Bader Lange, M.L., Sultana, R. and Butterfield, D.A. "Nutritional Approaches to Modulate Oxidative Stress in Alzheimer's Disease." Current Alzheimer Research 8, no. 5: 452 (2011)

Ringman, J.M., et al. "A Potential Role of the Curry Spice Curcumin in Alzheimer's Disease." Current Alzheimer Research 2, no. 2: 131–36 (2005)

Lautenschlager, N.T., Cox, K.L., Flicker, L., Foster, J.K., Frank, P., van Bockxmeer, M., Xiao, J. Greenop, K.R., Almeida, O.P. "Effect of Physical Activity on Cognitive Function in Older Adults at Risk for Alzheimer Disease: A Randomized Trial." The Journal of the American Medical Association: 97 (2008)

Cédric Annweiler, Yves Rolland, Anne M Schott, Hubert Blain, Bruno Vellas, François R Herrmann, and Olivier Beauchet. "Higher Vitamin D Dietary Intake Is Associated With Lower Risk of Alzheimer's Disease: A 7-Year Follow-up." Journal of Gerontology: MEDICAL SCIENCES (March 7, 2012)

The Alzheimer's Prevention Cookbook: Recipes to Boost Brain Health. Ten Speed Press, Berkeley, CA (2012)

## Chapter 15

Medical News Today. "Alternatives To Nursing Homes—How To Improve Seniors Quality Of Life." http://www.medicalnewstoday.com/articles/247332.php (2012)

Morgan, M. Your Health, The Nation, and the Senior Healthcare System. BodyEnergy Company DVD (2014)

Medicare.gov. "Nursing Homes: Alternatives to Nursing Home Care." www.medicare.gov/nursing/alternatives.asp (2012)

Pennsylvania Department of Public Health. "Alternatives to Nursing Homes." www.dpw.state.pa.us/fordisabilityservices/alternativestonursinghomes/index.htm (2014)

De Beauvoir, Simone. The Coming of Age.  Editions Gallimard (1972)

Thomas, Bill. "Changing Aging." www.changingaging.org (2014)

AARP Foundation. "Navigating the world of caregiving." http://assets.aarp.org/external_sites/caregiving/index.html (2014)